Running Injuries

How to prevent and overcome them

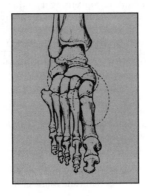

Tim Noakes
Stephen Granger

Cape Town
Oxford University Press
1996

OXFORD UNIVERSITY PRESS
Walton Street, Oxford OX2 6DP, United Kingdom

Oxford   New York
Athens   Bangkok   Bombay
Calcutta   Cape Town   Dar es Salaam   Delhi
Florence   Hong Kong   Istanbul   Karachi
Kuala Lumpur   Madras   Madrid   Melbourne
Mexico City   Nairobi   Paris   Singapore
Taipei   Tokyo   Toronto

and associated companies in
Berlin   Ibadan

OXFORD is the trade mark of Oxford University Press

RUNNING INJURIES
ISBN 0 19 571384 2

First published 1990
Second edition 1996
© Oxford University Press Southern Africa 1990, 1996

Commissioning editors: Hanri Pieterse and Helen Laurenson
Editors: Helen Laurenson and Angela Briggs
Designer: Mara Singer (based on an original design by New Leaf Design)
Cover design: Mara Singer
Illustrations: Jeanette Venter
Index: Sandie Vahl
Photographs: Stephen Granger and Touchline Photo (pp 9, 29, 59, 87, 107)
Cover photographs: Touchline Photo, Image Bank and Mark Standley

Published by Oxford University Press Southern Africa
Harrington House, Barrack Street, Cape Town 8001, South Africa

Set in 9 on 11½ pt Stone Serif by Photoprint
Reproduction by Photoprint
Cover reproduction by Photoprint
Printed and bound by ABC Book Printers, Kinghall Avenue, Epping Industria II

Acknowledgements
We are grateful to all the runners who contributed to this book by sharing their personal experiences of injury. Particular thanks are due to Soulman Nakedi and Tanya Peckham, who posed for several photographs. The running stride photographs in Chapter 2 are based on diagrams devised by S I Subotnik (*Podiatric Sports Medicine*, Futura Publishing Company, New York).

A letter to our readers

Tim Noakes

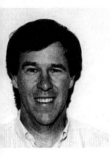

Stephen Granger

Most runners find themselves injured, in pain, or even laid off, at some time in their running careers. This happens despite the fact that there is a growing body of knowledge about the treatment and prevention of running injuries. When we wrote *Running Injuries* in 1990, we did so because it seemed to us that runners needed access to this information. It was our hope that the book would help hundreds of resurrected sportspeople to return to vigorous exercise in the shortest possible time.

At that time we felt that runners needed to understand not only the cause of their injury, but how to get the best possible treatment for it. In this edition, we hope to add to this by focusing on how to avoid injury in the first place — running without injury must always be better than recovery. So we have expanded chapter 4 — *Prevention is better than cure* — and have also included a discussion of factors that predispose to injury, and a quick checklist for practising injury-free running.

One of the best sources of information about what works and what doesn't are runners themselves. In this updated edition, elite South African and international runners give practical advice on how to stay injury-free. Having spoken to these runners, we are convinced that preventing injury is one of the most important ways of achieving your athletic goals.

However, runners do become injured and so we have also included in this edition the most up-to-date insights from sports science on treating injury, particularly in *A troubleshooter's guide*. Again, elite athletes describe their injuries and relate how they overcame them.

A new glossary and index should make the information in *Running Injuries* even more quickly accessible to runners of all levels.

Tim Noakes and Stephen Granger

Contents

1 New insights into running injuries

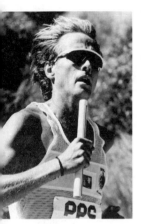

The revolution in the understanding of running injuries

There are two kinds of sports injuries. Some result from the application of a single, irresistible force to the body and cause the immediate onset of pain and disability. These injuries are classified as extrinsic injuries and occur especially in contact or collision-type sports like rugby, soccer or boxing.

Extrinsic injuries are traditionally well catered for by medicine. After all, trauma is a natural component of our society and many people not involved in sport suffer injuries that are no different from those experienced by the modern gladiators.

In contrast, intrinsic injuries do not originate from forces outside the body and their onset is typically gradual. Characteristic intrinsic injuries are found in long distance runners. Before the early 1970s, the methods used for treating running injuries were the same as those used for treating traumatic injuries. The possibility that these injuries were the result of other mechanisms was not seriously considered. The result was that few of these injuries were effectively treated and runners with chronic injuries usually became non-runners. The best treatment that the experts were able to prescribe for injured runners was rest, physiotherapy, drugs and, if all else failed, surgery. Unfortunately, all else did usually fail and surgery was seldom any more successful.

Then, in the early 1970s, a group of American podiatrists including Dr Richard Schuster and Dr Steven Subotnik, aided by a marathon-running cardiologist, Dr George Sheehan, started to promote the concept that there was a missing X-factor in these injuries. It soon became apparent that these injuries resulted from the interaction of three factors: the genetics of the athlete, the environment in which training was done, and the athlete's training methods. It was necessary to correct all three if the injury was to be prevented or cured.

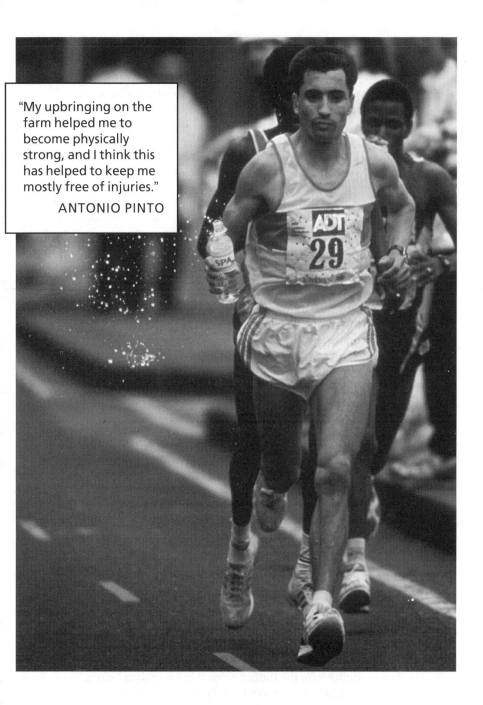

"My upbringing on the farm helped me to become physically strong, and I think this has helped to keep me mostly free of injuries."

ANTONIO PINTO

Possibly one of the most useful cases in prompting these new insights was that of a tough-minded United States ex-marine. Severe knee pain had proved insufficient to put a stop to his running career although it had proved resistant to every therapeutic intervention that Sheehan or anyone else had prescribed. He was finally saved when he developed foot pain in addition to his knee injury and was referred to a foot specialist. The in-shoe foot support (corrective orthotic) that was prescribed to relieve the foot pain, cured not only that injury but also his knee pain.

From this fortuitous event, Sheehan and the podiatrists drew the empirical conclusion that the runner's foot problem might have something to do with other running injuries in other parts of the anatomy. This heralded a new era in the understanding of running injuries.

Through his daily contact with injured runners, Sheehan observed further cases which suggested that the traditional approach to running injuries might be inadequate. For example, a high school runner told him that his knees hurt only when he trained in a particular pair of shoes. Another suffered pain only when he ran in one direction continuously on a banked track. Sheehan himself found that he experienced pain when running on one side of a cambered road, although he was pain-free when running on the opposite side.

These were among the first attempts (whether conscious or not) to move the discipline of running injuries outside the field of conventional medicine, especially orthopaedic surgery. Understanding running injuries had become more a logical thought process based on a knowledge of the mechanics of running and the history of the injured runner, than a dependency on sophisticated medical resources. Knowledge of the structure of the lower limb and of materials used in the manufacture of running shoes became of more benefit to the injured runners than expertise related to drugs which might be optimistically injected into some part of the injured runner's anatomy.

New hope for the injured runner

Since the first new insights of the 1970s, the understanding of running injuries has become much more sophisticated. The outlook for the runner is much brighter than before.

What is of concern is the epidemic of running injuries — the modern day athletic pandemic. What makes running injuries so dangerous is that doctors often fail to think about the root cause, and so treatment fails. Running injuries have a unique feature: an identifiable and treatable cause. And until that cause is rectified, the conventional approach — the rest, the drugs, the injections and surgery — is (as Sheehan showed in the seventies) just an expensive waste of time.

Hopefully this book will go some way towards redressing the failures of the past. We trust that it will provide runners with an understanding of how their own genetic predispositions make them vulnerable to injury; with the means to remain injury-free; and, where they are already injured, with the hope of returning to their chosen sport in the shortest possible time.

2 Understanding the body

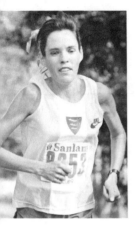

The biomechanics of body motion

The physical laws which govern the mechanics of body motion are somewhat complex and certainly beyond the understanding of the authors of this book. So we shall leave the understanding of such concepts to physicists, mathematicians and engineers — experts better able than we to cope with the mathematical formulae governing the forces acting on the intricate moving object that is a runner. But a knowledge of the basic principles of the mechanics of running is essential for understanding why runners become injured; and fortunately, these fundamental principles are rather more accessible.

Basic principles of the ideal running stride

The running stride
The running stride is divided into two major phases, the support or stance phase (during which the foot is in contact with the ground) and the longer swing or recovery phase. The heelstrike of one foot to the next heelstrike of the same foot makes up one running cycle. In other words, two running strides make up one running cycle. During each running stride, the leg rotates in the following sequence (see photograph sequence beginning on page 14).

The ankle as a universal joint
As soon as the foot is planted on the ground (position 12), the frictional forces between the sole and the surface of the ground prevent the foot from passively following the internal/external rotation sequence occurring in the lower limb. Therefore a mechanism is present that allows the rotation sequence of the upper limb to continue without involving actual movement of the foot in relation to the ground.

To achieve this, the joint just below the ankle, the subtalar joint, acts as a universal joint, transmitting the internal rotation

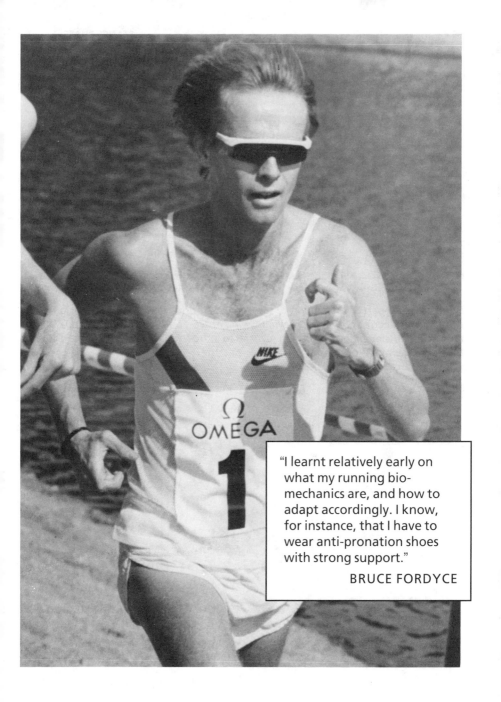

"I learnt relatively early on what my running bio-mechanics are, and how to adapt accordingly. I know, for instance, that I have to wear anti-pronation shoes with strong support."

BRUCE FORDYCE

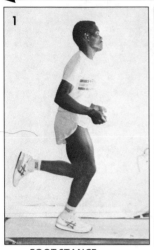 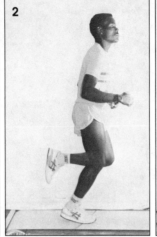 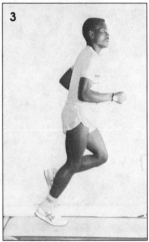

FOOT STANCE   MID-SUPPORT

During the first part of the support or stance phase (position 1) an inward rotation of the leg, which began during the previous swing phase, continues. By mid-support (position 2), the direction of rotation reverses to one of outward (external) rotation and this continues at toe-off (positions 3 to 4).

SWING PHASE

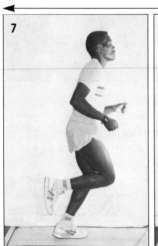 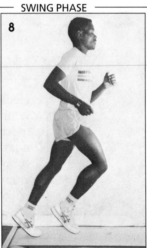 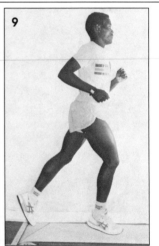

FORWARD SWING

This rotation continues during the latter part of the swing phase. The big toe moves towards the midline of the body during this rotation.

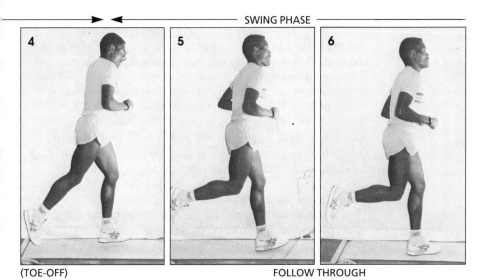

(TOE-OFF)   FOLLOW THROUGH

Immediately after toe-off, during the longer swing or recovery phase of the cycle, the leg begins to rotate inwards (positions 5 to 11).

SWING PHASE   STANCE PHASE

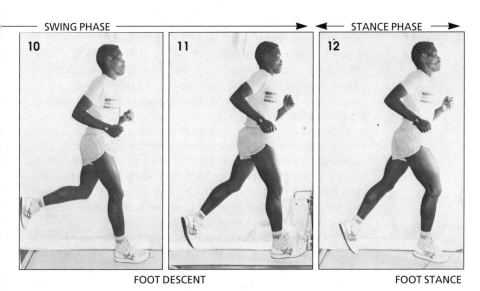

FOOT DESCENT   FOOT STANCE

Top Cape Town road athlete, Soulman Nakedi, demonstrates the running stride on the treadmill of the MRC/UCT Bioenergetics of Exercise Research Unit. The labels refer to the action of the right leg only. Note that the actual position of toe-off for the right foot is not shown in the photographs. Left foot toe-off can be seen in position 8.

of the lower limb (in the transverse plane) into an inward rolling or pronatory movement at the ankle (in the frontal or horizontal plane). In this way the rotational plane moves through ninety degrees.

As the ankle joint pronates, it unlocks the joints of the midfoot, allowing these also to roll inward. These joint movements are collectively known as pronation. Pronation is accompanied by a lowering of the arch and increased flexibility of the foot, enabling the foot to absorb and distribute the shock of landing and to adapt to an uneven running surface.

'Normal' or 'ideal' gait

In the athlete with normal running mechanics, after fifty-five to sixty percent of the stance phase has been completed, the upper limb begins to rotate externally (outwards). The ankle rotation reverses itself and rotation now occurs outwards (this is known as supination). Then, just before toe-off, the ankle and midfoot joints lock in a fully supinated position. This results in the lower limb becoming a rigid lever, allowing for a powerful toe-off.

In the ideal running gait there is an early, limited degree of pronation near the beginning of the stance phase. This is followed some time near the middle of the stance phase of the running stride, by supination of the subtalar joint.

In other words, during the period of contact with the ground the ideal foot transforms from a mobile adapter to a rigid lever. At some point between the two extremes a neutral position is achieved, where the joints and bones are perfectly aligned for optimum function.

Unfortunately, only a very small percentage of runners have a sufficiently normal biomechanical structure to allow this normal sequence of events. Most of us are saddled with feet that either do too much rolling (the hypermobile foot) or else roll too little (the rigid or 'clunk' foot). And when feet are attached to minor malalignments in the lower limb, it becomes remarkable that any runner can escape injury.

Another important concept is the length of running stride. It is important that the foot should land directly under the centre of gravity of the body. In the swing phase the foot swings forward and then begins swinging back (positions 5 to 11) and lands as the body catches up with the foot (position 12). The key is that it should do so at zero acceleration under the body's centre of gravity. If a runner attempts to change this through

Bruce Fordyce *(South Africa)*

Possibly the world's greatest ever ultra-marathon athlete. Began running at twenty while studying archaeology at Wits University. Unparalleled record in Comrades Marathon (86 km – 89 km). Placed 43rd, 14th, third, and second, thereafter winning eight successive races between 1981 and 1988. Won a 100 km race in Stellenbosch in February 1989 in 6:25:07 against many of the world's top 100 km athletes. Ninth Comrades win in 1990. Holds both the 'up' record (5:27:42) and the 'down' (5:24:07). Successive wins at 86 km London to Brighton between 1981 and 1983. His 5:12:32 record in 1983 included a world best for 50 miles of 4:50:21, which remains unsurpassed and which is 31 minutes faster than the world 50 mile track record (1995). American 80 km record of 4:50:50 in the American Medical Joggers Association (AMJA) 80 km Marathon in 1987. Won the 1987 Nanisivik Midnight Sun 84 km Marathon in the Arctic Circle in record time (6:33:00). Best standard marathon time of 2:17:18, set in East London in 1983.

Interview

I learnt relatively early on what my running biomechanics are, and how to adapt accordingly. I know, for instance, that I have to wear anti-pronation shoes with strong support. I sometimes feel a slight niggling pain starting to come on in my calves and I know that the mid-sole of my shoe has collapsed — even if it is only by millimetres. A change of shoes is usually all that is required.

overstriding (foot lands in front of centre of gravity) or understriding (foot lands behind centre of gravity), not only will the runner's shoes wear out more quickly, but injury could also result.

How our structural realities interfere with the ideal running stride

We have learned how an ex-marine was cured of his knee pain when he sought treatment for an injured foot. In the years since those first therapeutic miracles were effected in the seventies, Sheehan and his podiatric colleagues have taught us that the key to the successful treatment of running injuries is to be on the lookout for that mysterious X-factor, that hidden factor responsible for the runner's injury.

We have learned that those very ingredients that make athletes great — genetic endowment, training methods and training environment — are the same factors responsible for their injuries. There are a myriad in-built afflictions, each a potential destroyer — ranging from the internal twist of the femur or tibia, the squinting patellae, the bow legs or knock-knees, to the short leg and the flat or high-arched.

When these genetic factors are exposed to the hostile environment of shoes and surfaces and are expected to withstand impossible training loads, injury becomes not only possible, but inevitable. Treatment of the injury must take into account every possible contributory factor — the genetics, the environment and the training.

The critical genetic factor that predisposes to running injuries is lower limb structure because this largely determines how our hips, knees and ankles and their supporting structures — muscles, tendons and ligaments — function during running. Because of differences in genetic structure, virtually no two runners function identically. More importantly, perfect mechanical function is exceedingly rare and is restricted to a handful of top runners. The rest of us run despite varying grades of biomechanical disaster.

The description in the early 1970s of the way in which these structural abnormalities interfere with the normal functioning of the foot and lower limb during running — and how they interact with running surfaces, shoes and training methods — was probably the most important recent advance in sports medicine. Although the phenomenon is not yet fully understood, it seems there is a common pathway by which these abnormalities cause running injuries. For example, we have seen that in 'normal' gait the foot doubles as a pronator to dissipate impact shock waves and as a supinator to provide a rigid lever for toe-off. Unfortunately structural abnormalities leave some runners short on pronation and others short on supination, predisposing each group to specific types of injuries, which are discussed in the remainder of this chapter.

If we are to develop a better understanding of the reason for our injuries and so determine the most effective means of overcoming them, we must examine the most important lower limb abnormalities.

Structural deficiencies

The list of genetic afflictions that can predispose to running injuries includes: leg-length asymmetry (short leg syndrome), genu varum (bow legs), genu valgum (knock knees), forefoot or rearfoot malalignment, twisting (internal rotation) of the femur, externally (outwardly) or internally (inwardly) rotated tibia, squinting or 'kissing' patella, high-arched feet and flat feet.

In fairly broad terms, the lower limb mechanics of injured runners usually exhibit one of two characteristic patterns — either the foot rotates inward (pronates) too much, or it does not pronate enough. The foot that rotates too little is almost always the 'clunk' (high-arched) foot, whereas the foot that pronates too much is referred to as hypermobile, flexible or simply flat.

A popular method for identifying a flexible or rigid foot is the 'bathroom test'. Place your still-wet foot on the bath mat first when you are sitting, then when you are standing. The imprint of most runners will look like imprint 2 in the photograph on this page when they are sitting. If the standing foot imprint looks like imprint 3, the runner has a rigid ('clunk') foot, while imprint 1 is that of a flat (hypermobile) foot. The same test can be performed standing on wet sand. The importance of identifying the foot type is that foot types 1 and 3 cause injuries for different reasons.

The 'clunk' foot
The 'clunk' foot is a rigid, stable, immobile, high-arched structure that is unable to perform the most basic functions of

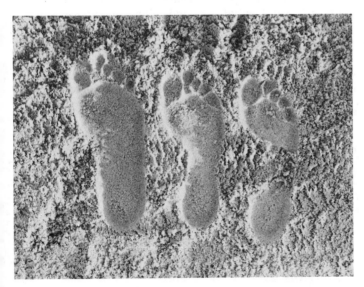

Footprints in the sand: the telltale signs. The imprint on the left (1) is that of a flat foot, the one in the centre (2) corresponds with a normal foot, and the imprint on the right (3) is that of a high-arched rigid foot.

the running foot — adequate shock absorption through controlled, appropriate pronation. Because of its stability, the 'clunk' foot provides a powerful lever at push-off and so is the ideal foot for the sprinter. But in long-distance running in which adequate shock absorption is essential, particularly during days of heavy training or in a long race when fatigued muscles lose their ability to absorb shock, the clunker is a major source of disaster. So much so, that a good percentage, possibly thirty to forty percent, of injured runners have this type of foot. As the high-arched foot is unable to absorb sufficient shock, it places additional stresses on other shock-absorbing structures, particularly in the foot (the achilles tendon and the plantar fascia) and around the knee, which may break down.

Injuries associated with this foot include stress fractures, iliotibial band syndrome, trochanteric bursitis and ill-defined muscle and joint pain. Achilles tendonitis and plantar fasciitis may also be caused by this foot type. (This does not necessarily conflict with the possibility that pronation can also cause these injuries.)

The hypermobile foot
This foot is an excellent shock-absorber because of its ability to pronate, but it is very unstable during the push-off phase of running. Instead of having a firm lever from which to push off, the runner with the hypermobile foot is all but attached to the ground by a bag of delinquent bones, each going its own way and causing the lower limb to rotate too far inwards during the stance phase of running. It is this excessive inward rotation that causes the most common injuries. The classic injuries associated with this foot are peripatellar pain syndrome ('runner's knee') and popliteus tendonitis, but plantar fasciitis, achilles tendonitis, tibial or fibular bone strain ('shinsplints') and stress fractures can also occur in this foot type.

The inbetweener
In between these two types of running feet, there is an intermediate foot which combines the weaknesses of both. Not only is the foot high-arched, but it is also malaligned. It combines just enough rigidity with just too much motion so that the medicine that works for either of the other foot types may be useless for this type. Another danger inherent in this foot type is that if its pronation is too well controlled with appropriate shoes and corrective orthotics, the original injury may be cured, but

another injury may be caused because the foot can no longer absorb shock adequately.

Other structural defects

Although we have considered here only foot abnormalities, other structural defects can exacerbate the problem and delay the return of injured runners to the uninhibited enjoyment of their sport.

For example, the foot of the person with bow legs may use its full range of pronation simply to allow the border of the foot to reach the ground just when standing. When running, the foot may therefore be unable to pronate further and will thus become an inadequate shock absorber. Thus the combination of bow legs and a high-arched foot compounds the likelihood of an injury owing to impaired shock absorption.

The Q angle or quadriceps angle is used to indicate the presence of a structural abnormality which causes the kneecap, or patella, to drift inwards during the stance phase of running. The Q angle is the angle between the line connecting the centre of the kneecap to the anterior iliac spine on the pelvis, and the line connecting the tibial tuberosity and the centre of the kneecap, as shown in the diagram below. Runners with a Q angle greater than sixteen degrees are at significantly increased risk of developing runner's knee.

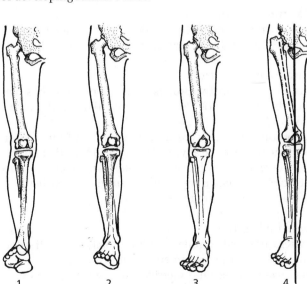

The Q angle affects the running stride.

1. Contact
2. Pronates
3. Lower leg twists inward
4. Q angle

3 Understanding the mind

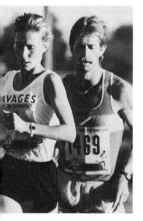

The influence of the mind

We have gained considerable insight over the past fifteen years into the cause of injury through learning to understand the body better. But we are now discovering that there are other factors which limit our effectiveness in treating some runners. We are realizing that the newer, now conventional remedies, cure the majority of runners but are quite useless in some. They are useless because, like a good percentage of ordinary medical patients, some runners can never get better. Their problem is more a mental than a physical one — perhaps it could be termed excessive pronation of the brain.

Psychological factors determining an athlete's response to injury

Personal factors

Certain factors influence how athletes will interact both with their injury and with the person they consult about their injury.

Desire to be in control

There are essentially two groups of injured runners: those who wish to be in control of their treatment and those who wish to be controlled.

Obviously their needs are quite different. The former require little more than simple advice of the type provided in this book. The latter require very precise and detailed instructions and are likely to recover only if they can find an adviser capable of helping them in this way.

Level of self-esteem

Athletes whose self-confidence is low usually require the doctor to take charge of their treatment. If left to do things by themselves they become excessively stressed and anxious.

The opposite extreme is the athlete whose level of self-

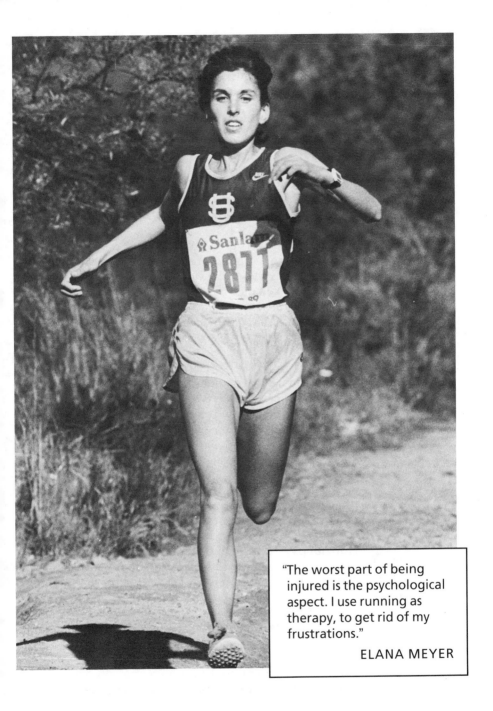

"The worst part of being injured is the psychological aspect. I use running as therapy, to get rid of my frustrations."

ELANA MEYER

confidence is too high, frequently unjustifiably so. Such athletes find it difficult to trust and listen to the opinions of others. They have unshakeable confidence in their own way of doing things and know better than their doctors how to solve their medical problems. Under pressure, this tendency often increases. All doctors will have difficulty with this type of athlete.

Speed of decision-making
People differ in the speed at which they make decisions and may react differently to doctors whose speed of decision-making differs from their own.

Degree of extroversion–introversion
Quiet, introverted athletes become even more so when injured and it is often extremely difficult to extract all the necessary information about their injury from them. In contrast, the extroverted athlete may use denial and joking to avoid facing the reality of the injury. This approach will pose a problem if it prevents the athlete from facing up to the seriousness of the injury.

Interpersonal expressiveness
The way we express ourselves has an intellectual and an emotional component and the amount of importance we attach to either will differ. For some there is a tendency to be logical and rational ('left brain dominant' behaviour). When such an athlete is injured, a structured treatment protocol will be better received than understanding and commiseration. Others, who are 'right-brain dominant', may express themselves more through emotions, which might be positive and supportive, negative and critical, or confrontational.

Normal psychological patterns of response to injury
Regardless of personality, athletes will go through a typical pattern of response to injury.

The stage of denial
At first, the athlete refuses to accept the reality of the injury and simply denies the possibility of a genuine problem.

The stage of anger (rage)
When the injury can no longer be denied, the athlete becomes

Elana Meyer *(South Africa)*

Born in October 1966 on a farm near Albertina, about 300 km east of Cape Town, she has emerged as SA's best-ever distance athlete. SA's second best (behind Zola Pieterse) over 1500 m (4:02:15), and best over 3000 m (8:32:00), 5000 m (14:44:15), and 10 000 m (30:52:51) on the track, and 10 km (31:33), 15 km (46:57), 21 km (67:22), and 42 km (2:25:15) on the road. World's best over 15 km (46:57) in Cape Town in 1991. Won 1993 Tokyo Half-Marathon in 67:22.

Marathon best of 2:25:15 in placing third at Boston in 1994. Finished second at Boston in 1995 in 2:26:51. Olympic silver medal in 10 000 m in 1992, Commonwealth silver medal in 10 000 m in 1994, World Cup gold medal in 10 000 m in 1994, and World Half-Marathon gold medal in 1994. Sixth in World Cross-Country Championships in both 1993 and 1994. Fifth in 10 000 m at the 1995 World Track Championships.

Interview
The worst part of being injured is the psychological aspect. I use running as therapy, to get rid of my frustrations and energy. I became very restless and frustrated during my enforced lay-off in 1989 (see page 135). I enjoy the freedom associated with running but then the pain prevented me from relishing that experience.

I have learnt to be more cautious in my approach to racing. I now rest far more both before and after a hard race to enable my body to recover.

---

enraged and blames either the doctor or some third party for the injury. Occasionally the body will be blamed for this 'betrayal' and may even be subjected to further abuse.

The stage of depression
When denial and rage no longer work, the stage of depression sets in.

The stage of acceptance
Finally, after some months, the athlete learns to accept the injury and to modify ambition to accommodate the inadequacies of the mortal body. When this occurs the runner is likely to be over the injury.

But a real problem is that acceptance of mortality frequently lasts only as long as the injury. Once the injury has healed, the athlete forgets the promises made when injured.

Some specific psychological injury patterns

The Munchausen syndrome

Baron von Munchausen lived in Hanover in the mid-eighteenth century and achieved notoriety as a teller of extraordinary tales about his life as a soldier in the Russian army and as a hunter and sportsman. The connection of Munchausen's name to a medical condition was made by Dr Richard Asher, who described a group of patients who were so addicted to surgery that they learnt to tell detailed, very appropriate, but totally untrue stories about their imagined illnesses. In this way, they fooled the surgeons into believing they desperately needed whichever surgical operation they desired.

The Munchausens are probably excessively rare amongst runners. Yet there are a few runners whose love of running is, one suspects, exceeded only by their love of surgery.

The runner who does not want to get better

A variant of the Munchausen syndrome is the runner who has to have a (simulated) injury which is, and always will be, incurable, surgery or no surgery. Such patients have dependant personalities and use their simulated illnesses either to avoid work or family responsibilities or to gain attention and sympathy. A variant of this injury is the psyche-out injury.

The iatrogenic injury syndrome

'Iatrogenic' is the Greek for doctor-induced. And there are a number of ways in which doctors, either alone or in combination, can ensure that certain running injuries never heal.

First is the situation in which the runner with a real injury suffers the misfortune of being shunted from one doctor to another without ever getting better. The runner soon concludes, or is told openly, that the injury is incurable and that it will be impossible ever to run again. This advice is usually incorrect.

Another type of iatrogenic injury is induced by society, not by doctors. It occurs when particular social norms which govern the society in which the injured runner lives, suggest that running, for whatever reason, may not be an acceptable pastime. This attitude, prevalent in the 1960s and 1970s, has largely disappeared, thanks especially in South Africa to the heroic performances of athletes like Bruce Fordyce, Mathews Temane and Frith van der Merwe.

The psyche-out injury syndrome (injury as an escape)

This is one of the most common psychological running injuries. In these cases, the runner uses injury either to explain a poor performance or to prevent a good performance.

Another variant is the runner who becomes psychologically injured shortly before an extreme event such as an ultra-marathon. These runners lack the psychological mechanisms to cope with these longer races and are best encouraged to stick to the shorter distances. There is no disgrace in being scared of over-extending oneself.

The over-eager parent syndrome (injury as a weapon)

Unfortunately, some parents never understand that participation in sport should always be to the principal benefit of the participant. They believe that their children participate in sport purely to fulfil their own (displaced) parental desires. When such parents 'push' their offspring in ways unacceptable to the child, the child may choose injury as a way of escape.

By being 'injured', the reluctant athlete achieves several objectives: making the parent feel guilty for pressurizing behaviour, frustrating the parent's misplaced aspirations and avoiding the undesired competition.

Two pointers that make the diagnosis very likely are the overbearing presence of a parent whose desire for the child's success is clearly abnormal and the extreme reluctance of the 'injured' athlete even to try participating in the sport. In contrast, the athlete with a real injury cannot wait to return to his or her favourite sport, and must be actively restrained!

The 'my-injury-is-unique' syndrome

Runners with this syndrome are usually outwardly intelligent and successful people. They usually contend that their injury is unique and that their doctor will almost certainly know nothing about it. These runners usually exude some hostility.

Another variant of this syndrome is the runner who vehemently accuses the doctor of causing the injury, either because of something the doctor wrote, or failed to write, or because of something someone said the doctor had said or written.

In conclusion Understanding the psychology of injury gives one an understanding of the medical approach that will be most likely to get our bodies or minds over the injury.

4 Prevention is better than cure

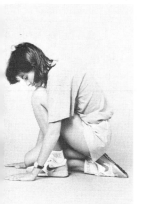

Guarding against injury

It is important to understand why runners become injured and to diagnose and treat injuries successfully. But it would be far better had these injuries not occurred in the first place. There are a number of factors associated with a higher risk of injury. It is important to understand these factors and adapt to accommodate them:

Gender
Women have wider hips and are therefore more likely to have biomechanical abnormalities in the lower limbs that predispose to injury. Women who restrict their energy intake to such an extent that they suffer menstrual disturbances can develop osteoporosis. This increases the risk of a bone injury such as a stress fracture.

Anatomical abnormalities of the lower limb
The anatomical abnormalities that predispose to running injuries were described in Chapter 2. Runners with these structural weaknesses need to approach their running with greater care.

Heavy weight
Overweight runners experience increased loading on the lower limbs and back during running. They are thus more likely to develop osteoarthritis of the knees and hips than runners who are the ideal body weight.

Inflexibility
Inflexibility of the muscles of the lower limb, especially the calf, hamstrings and quadriceps muscle groups and the iliotibial band, may also contribute to injury.

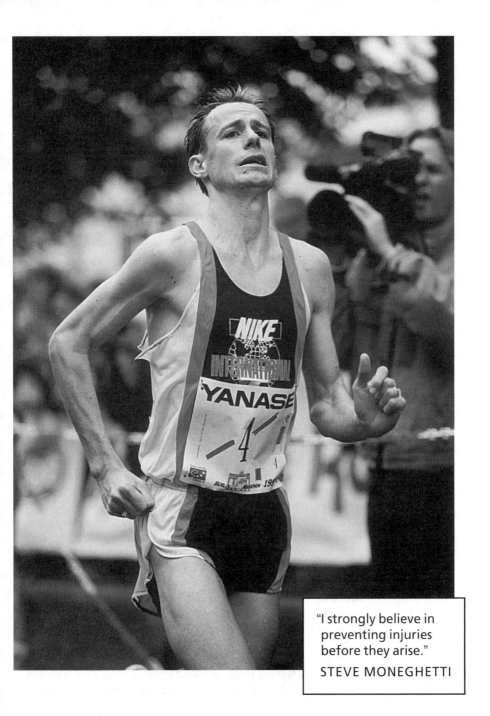

"I strongly believe in preventing injuries before they arise."

STEVE MONEGHETTI

Training

Finally, a number of factors associated with training can increase one's chances of being injured. These will be discussed in more detail below.

Staying injury-free

Keeping these factors in mind, there are three crucial considerations for remaining injury-free. These are an appropriate training programme on surfaces suited to our biomechanical requirements; the selection of shoes that will accommodate and compensate for our structural abnormalities; and a custom-built stretching programme to maintain muscle flexibility.

Training methods

How much? How fast?

There is no magic formula for athletes to determine the maximum weekly training distance or number of speed sessions possible before risking breakdown owing to injury. This will vary not only according to each athlete (and hence each set of biomechanical variables) but also according to the different phases in a particular athlete's career.

A critical point to understand is that it is not necessary to train to the point of breakdown in order to achieve optimum performance. Injury always means that the training load is too high. This is why injury frequently follows a sudden increase in training distance or speed (training too much, too fast, too soon, too frequently). This kind of injury also occurs when too many races or long runs have been undertaken, when the total training load has been too severe for too long, or when leg muscles have not recovered fully from a previous training session. The high school track athlete syndrome is a classic example. Following a long off-season, the enthusiastic athlete is subjected to an inordinately intensive training regime in order to peak for the first track meeting (see bone strain page 121). Unfortunately, this pattern is reflected in the approach of many distance runners. For whatever reason, these runners are unable or unwilling to adopt a more conservative, longer-term approach to their training and frequently pay the inevitable price.

Similarly, runners are at risk during the period where their bones are adapting to an increased training load. Typically this is eight to twelve weeks after the start of a training programme

Eamonn Martin *(United Kingdom)*

Raced competitively from early years. Won national under fifteen cross-country title in 1973 and the under seventeen 1500 m title in 1975, before winning senior titles in 1984 and 1992. Holder of British 10 000 m record (27:23:06) in 1988 and won gold medal in the 10 000 m at the 1990 Commonwealth Games in 28:08:57. 5000 m personal best of 13:20:94 (1983). Won the London Marathon in 1993 in 2:10:50 (PB), finished eighth in 1994 (2:11:05) and 13th in 1995 (2:12:44). Won 1995 Chicago Marathon in 2:11:18. Has represented his country in track, cross-country and on the road.

Interview

I guess I'm pretty injury-prone and have struggled through several injuries. But I have kept my injuries to a minimum since 1986 through exercises and preventative measures.

Since I had achilles surgery in 1987, I've made it a habit to consult my podiatrist every year for an analysis of any biomechanical changes and to check out my orthotics. I wear soft orthotics, which need to be replaced regularly, and hard orthotics in my casual shoes.

In addition, I see an osteopath once a week. He checks my back structure and works on posture, tight muscles and any muscle imbalances. I also try to fit in a massage about once a week, especially when I'm building up to a race.

I stretch for about twenty to thirty minutes before each run, as part of the warm-up session, but do not stretch after the run.

(either from scratch as a novice runner or following a long lay-off). At this point the cardiovascular fitness of the runner has increased to a level where harder training is possible. However, at the same time, the resorption process (see stress fractures page 68) has resulted in the runner's bones being at their weakest.

We have seen that muscle inflexibility is a factor in causing injuries. Muscles are likely to be relatively inflexible in the early morning, indicating a possible increased risk during this time.

A runner's history of training and injury will be a good indication of what (in terms of how much and how fast) is a manageable training and racing load. This underlines the need to keep detailed log books as a record of how and why injuries occurred. Novices should be particularly cautious during the first three months and should err on the side of caution rather than greed. Runners who have been running for some time without injury have either followed sound advice in terms of their training programmes (and the other considerations covered in this chapter) or fall into that small category of fortunate runners with near-perfect genetic structure. Little they do or don't do is likely to result in an intrinsic injury.

In summary, it should be noted that the following factors could make an appreciable difference to the likelihood of injury due to inappropriate training methods:

Years of training
Bone injuries are frequently experienced by new runners starting a running programme or runners returning to training after a lay-off, especially where the training volume increases rapidly. These runners should start a training programme conservatively. On the other hand, veteran runners may be more at risk of persistent injuries such as chronic muscle injuries, achilles tendonitis, plantar fasciitis and osteitis pubis. These 'wear and tear' degenerative injuries are prevented by careful control of the amount of heavy training and racing undertaken.

Rate of progress
Progressing too rapidly — either at the start of a running career, or after a lay-off caused by injury — increases the risk of injury. Ideally, progress should be slow and allow the body the time it needs to adapt to the new demands.

Volume of weekly training
The frequency of injury rises with the volume of training done; but the rate of injury per kilometre run remains fairly constant. Thus, those who run a great deal are injured more simply because they run more kilometres and not because each successive kilometre they run becomes more risky.

Amount of speed training and racing
Speed training and racing increase the loading stresses on the body, increasing the risk of injury.

Time of day
Running in the early morning when the muscles are less flexible may increase injury risk. However, running in the early morning is usually done at a slower speed. This may counteract the increased risk of injury caused by inflexibility.

Colleen de Reuck *(South Africa)*

Started running at primary school about 200 km north of Durban. First road race (10 km) at fifteen and ran 1:16 half-marathon a year later. Won five SA Half-Marathon titles, between 1985 and 1989, beating Elana Meyer in 1989 with her best time of 68:38 — then third best in the world. 15 km PB of 48:19. Silver medal in SA Cross-Country Champion-ships behind Meyer in 1988, 1989, and 1991. 23rd in 1993 World Cross-Country Championships. 2:31:21 marathon debut in 1992 to qualify for Barcelona Olympics, where she placed eighth in 2:39:03. Moved to Boulder, Colorado in 1993. *Runner's World* Road Runner of the Year for 1993. Won 1993 Falmouth 7,1 mile and Philadelphia Half-Marathon. First child in 1994.

Interview   *Apart from a slight case of ITB while I was at university, until 1994 [see page 43] I had never really been injured.*

I think that I have been relatively injury-free for so long because I never train intensively through the year. I always include rest periods after intensive training. In addition I always make sure I wear shoes with good support during training. Although I wear lighter trainers for speed sessions, I never train in my racing shoes.

I often get stiff calves after races, probably because I run on my toes, but it's never really been a serious problem or prevented me from training.

Recovery between training sessions
Leg muscles that have not recovered fully from a previous training session are unable to absorb shock normally. As a result, the shock-absorbing role usually performed by the leg muscles must be taken over by the bones, ligaments and tendons of the lower limb, exposing those structures to an increased risk of injury.

Training during and after injury
Injury will always require an adaptation of one's training programme, at least in the short term, while rehabilitation is under way. This adaptation could be as radical as total rest in the case of stress fractures, but will more often take the form of 'modified rest' tailored to the grade of the injury (see page 58).

In general, as long as the injury remains in the first injury grade (pain only after exercise), it is probably not necessary to alter one's training programme dramatically. But for a grade II injury (pain coming on during exercise), it is advisable to reduce all speed running, particularly hill running, as well as racing, long runs and weekly training distance. When the injury reaches grade III (pain coming on during exercise and impairing performance), only short-distance jogging, cycling, swimming and 'running' in water with a flotation device are advised. Note that when 'running' in water, the athlete will be floating and there will be no foot contact with the bottom of the pool. With a grade IV injury (pain preventing running) there should be no normal running whatsoever. The only permissible activities are running in water, swimming and possibly cycling — and this last only in exceptional circumstances.

Running surfaces

Running surfaces are often too hard or too cambered. The ideal running surface is a soft, level surface such as a gravel road. Unfortunately, we are usually forced to run on tarred roads or concrete pavements. Furthermore, roads are usually cambered and this forces the foot on the higher part of the slope to rotate inwards (pronate) excessively, while the range of movement of the foot on the lower part of the slope is reduced. In addition, the leg on the lower side of the camber is artificially shortened and therefore acts as a 'short-leg'.

Grass surfaces, although soft, are uneven, while the sand on beaches is either too soft (above the high water mark) or too cambered (below the high water mark). Athletic tracks vary in hardness and introduce the problem of running continuously in one direction. This causes specific stresses on the outer leg, which must overstride to bring the athlete around each corner.

Similarly, uphill running puts the achilles tendon and calf muscles on the stretch and tilts the pelvis forward, while downhill running accentuates the impact shock of landing and pulls the pelvis backwards, thereby extending the back. Downhill running also causes the muscles to contract eccentrically (lengthen rather than shorten, owing to increased load) thereby increasing muscle damage. Overstriding, which is more common when running downhill, also increases the loading on the anterior calf muscles.

A running injury may first occur shortly after the athlete has changed to uphill or downhill running, or to running on the beach or on a synthetic or cinder track, or to running continuously on unfavourable road camber. Rather than stop running

Steve Moneghetti *(Australia)*

Began running at the age of fourteen in 1976. Lived all his life in Ballarat, near Melbourne, a scenic, forested town. First represented Australia as a junior in 1982 and as a senior at the World Cross-Country Championships in Lisbon in 1985, where he placed 101st. Has subsequently raced the World Cross-Country Championships on seven occasions, placing fourth in 1989 and sixth in 1992. Former world record holder for the half-marathon, having run 60:34 at the Great North Run in 1990. PB of 60:06 in Tokyo Half-Marathon in 1993 and placed second at World Half-Marathon Championships in that year. Marathon PB of 2:08:16 in winning at Berlin in 1990. Named *Athletics International* World No. 1 in the marathon for 1994 because of victories at Tokyo (2:08:55) and at the Commonwealth Games in Victoria.

Interview

I have a physical therapist who accompanies me to all my races and treats me before and after the event. I strongly believe in preventing injuries before they arise! I receive a massage at least once a week.

Another important factor is that at least ninety percent of my training is done off paved surfaces. It helps that I live in a part of the world blessed with many forest paths and other gravel roads. I think that limiting shock absorption where possible helps immeasurably.

I'm not really diligent about stretching. I do a bit before training runs, but it tends to be only about five or ten minutes.

Our comment

For an athlete who demands so much of himself, Moneghetti has suffered remarkably few injuries. He considers training on forest paths, and the preventative maintenance programme overseen by his physiotherapist, to be important factors in preventing injury.

for want of a perfect surface, it may be helpful to train on a variety of surfaces. If road camber is unavoidable, try to share the 'down' side equally between the right and left legs. If you are doing track work, do half the intervals running in one direction and the other half running in the opposite direction.

There is growing evidence that increased loading of the skeleton and muscles caused by, for example, running on hard surfaces in poorly cushioned shoes, is probably as important a factor in injuries as is excessive subtalar joint (ankle) pronation.

Shoes

Until very recently, running shoes were developed without attention to the possibility that they could cause running injuries. But now science and public demand have forced the running shoe manufacturers to produce shoes that will not only reduce the risk of injury, but will also cure injuries that already exist.

From the discussion on the biomechanics of running (page 12) it will be appreciated just how important the choice of the appropriate running shoes is for the different injuries and foot types. In particular, the two different foot types (high-arched or flat) and injury categories require quite opposite shoe characteristics to compensate for their inherent weaknesses.

Running shoes must therefore be designed either for adequate shock absorption or for motion control. These are two quite different characteristics which can be built into the same shoe only with great difficulty — because in general, the more a shoe is built for foot control, the more rigid it must be and consequently the less shock it can absorb. Conversely, the better the shock-absorbing capacity of the shoe, the less well it will control the foot. However, as we have said before, the importance of shock absorption may have been underestimated, even in injuries traditionally believed to result purely from excessive ankle pronation. Even runners who pronate severely should avoid excessively firm shoes. In all likelihood, these runners also need a shoe that will have reasonable shock-absorbing characteristics. The design of such shoes is now a major challenge for shoe manufacturers.

Shoes designed primarily for shock absorption

The following runners should wear these shoes:

☐ Runners who have bow legs
☐ Runners who have high-arched, rigid, 'clunk' feet
☐ Runners who suffer from, or who have suffered from
    — iliotibial band friction syndrome
    — stress fractures
    — trochanteric bursitis

The principle characteristic that makes a shoe soft enough to be acceptable for a rigid foot is a very soft mid-sole. Thus the EVA, air, gel or other component of the mid-sole will compress easily under firm thumb pressure. In addition, the heel-counter must

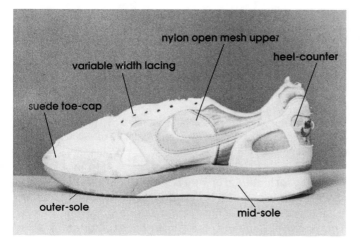

Features of a typical running shoe

nylon open mesh upper

variable width lacing

heel-counter

suede toe-cap

outer-sole

mid-sole

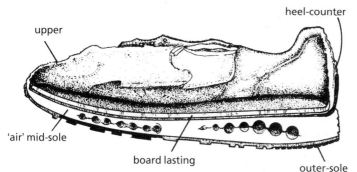

Features of a typical running shoe (bisected down the longitudinal axis)

heel-counter

upper

'air' mid-sole

board lasting

outer-sole

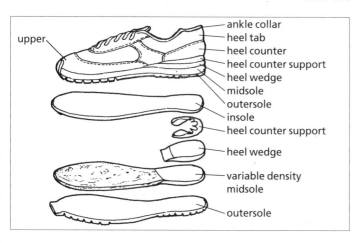

Components of a typical running shoe

upper

ankle collar
heel tab
heel counter
heel counter support
heel wedge
midsole
outersole
insole
heel counter support
heel wedge
variable density midsole
outersole

Catherina McKiernan *(Ireland)*

Born in County Cavan, the most consistent female cross-country athlete of the nineties. Won the international Cross Challenge Series competition four years in succession from 1992 and was four times silver medallist in the World Cross-Country Championships between 1992 and 1995, each time behind a different winner. Won European cross-country title in 1994. Beat Derartu Tulu and Elana Meyer in 10 000 m at Lille, France in June 1995. Personal bests of 31:19:11 for 10 000 m and 15:09:10 for 5000 m.

Interview *I have been fortunate to enjoy a relatively injury-free career and only in 1995 (see page 157) did injury curtail my racing career. Possibly because most of my training is done off paved surfaces, on grass, gravel, and sand roads, I have been spared many of the injuries often associated with top athletes. I have not trained extremely high mileages, and I think this has helped too. Generally I have stayed away from road racing, concentrating primarily on cross-country and track.*

be ineffective and should be made of a flexible, non-rigid material. A third characteristic of this shoe is that it should be slip-lasted and should not resist a twisting force applied along its long (vertical) axis.

Shoes designed primarily for foot control

The following runners should wear these shoes:

- ☐ Runners who have knock knees
- ☐ Runners who have hypermobile feet and who pronate excessively
- ☐ Runners who suffer from or who have suffered from
  - — peripatellar pain syndrome ('runner's knee')
  - — tibial or fibular bone strain ('shinsplints')
  - — achilles tendonitis
  - — plantar fasciitis

The features that increase a shoe's ability to resist pronation are obviously the exact opposite to those described above. Thus the anti-pronation shoe requires a mid-sole which is firm. Some manufacturers have increased selectively the firmness of the mid-sole material on the inner side of the shoe, which should resist the 'thumb compression test' (see page 40), with softer material on the sides. In addition, the shoe should be straight-lasted and must have a firm board last. The heel-counter must be rigid and durable. Another innovation introduced by some shoe manufacturers is to incorporate additional material that attaches the heel-counter more firmly to the mid-sole. This helps prevent separation of the heel-counter from the mid-sole, not an uncommon problem for runners who pronate excessively.

Corrective orthotics

For some runners who pronate excessively a strong anti-pronation shoe choice may not be enough to prevent or cure an injury. Corrective orthotics — arch supports specially made to remedy the individual athlete's problem — reduce both the total amount of rearfoot pronation and the maximum rate of pronation. This is compatible with the belief that orthotics can cure running injuries that are caused by excessive subtalar (ankle) joint pronation. Interestingly, corrective orthotics made of firm but soft material probably also increase shock absorption and this may also contribute to curing the injury. Firm plastic orthotics should not be used for running.

Monitoring shoes

Once shoes have been selected and bought, they should be carefully monitored to establish whether they are indeed appropriate for the specific biomechanical needs of the athlete. Anyone who continues to train normally but who becomes injured within two to four weeks after changing to a different running shoe, must consider that the new shoes could be the cause of the injury. In this case the treatment is obvious. Either go back to the old pair of running shoes or, if these are in bad repair, start running in a new pair of the same model.

It is also important to monitor shoes when they could be expected to be approaching the end of their 'life'. Incidentally, the life expectancy of shoes with EVA mid-soles is relatively short. As much as fifty percent of the shock-absorbing capacity of the EVA may be lost within six months with heavy use (400 km or more per month). The shock-absorbing capacity of shoes with air and gel mid-soles does not appear to alter with use. The only risk of these shoes is the development of a 'puncture'! Punctured shoes can unfortunately not be saved.

The major areas of failure in the running shoe are the heel-counter, the mid-sole and the outer-sole. The heel-counter may have lost its rigidity and may have been dragged inwards. This is

Running shoes of the supinator, showing severe wear of the outer-sole on the outer edge of each shoe

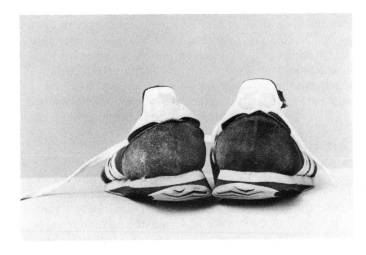

Section of running shoe showing collapsed mid-sole towards the inside of the shoe. Viewed towards the toe (left) and towards the heel (right)

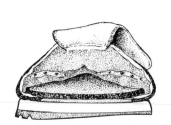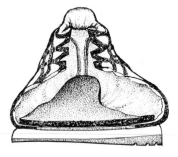

typical of athletes who pronate badly.

The mid-sole material in the heel is particularly prone to compaction, especially in running shoes in which the EVA mid-sole material is very soft. Uneven compaction can lead to imbalance in the heel, which can produce a running injury by itself. This illustrates the importance of checking one's shoes regularly from behind.

The mid-sole material in the forefoot can also compact, particularly in runners who land mainly on the balls of their feet, so-called forefoot strikers. The only way to detect this mid-sole compaction under the forefoot is to use the 'thumb compression test'. Put one hand inside the shoe and the other outside. Compare the mid-sole thickness at the point of greatest wear with the wear over the rest of the mid-sole by squeezing it between the fingers at different places.

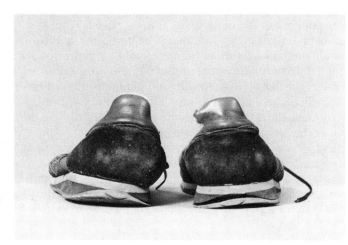

Running shoes of the extreme pronator. The heel-counters have been dragged inwards to a point where the wearer could almost be said to be running 'next to' the shoes

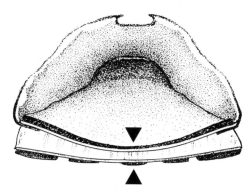

Running shoe in cross section showing compaction of mid-sole material under the forefoot

Most runners whose shoes have compacted front mid-soles will usually be aware of this because when they land on a stone underneath the forefoot, they feel immediate, sharp pain.

Finally, the mid-sole may have hardened or 'bottomed-out'. The 'thumb compression test' can be used to compare the relative hardness of the mid-sole of different running shoes. It can also reveal the degree to which a shoe has bottomed-out.

With experience you learn how much indentation corresponds to the exact softness or hardness of the shoe that is most appropriate for your needs.

Because shoes differ in the rapidity with which the mid-sole compacts or turns to 'stone', the test is also essential to check loss of shock absorbing capacity with time. If shock absorption is important to a particular athlete, then a marked loss of shock absorption may be sufficient to produce an injury.

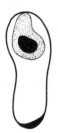

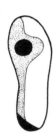

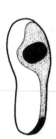

The last important area of shoe wear is the outer-sole. The diagram on the left shows the different wear patterns found in three different running styles. In the normal wear pattern (shoe on top), the outer-sole wears at the outer edge of the heel, under the ball of the foot between the first and second toes, and then at the front of the sole, underneath the second and third toes.

In contrast, the extreme pronator (middle shoe), strikes on the inside of the heel and wears all along the inside border of the sole and, in particular, underneath the big toe. The third type of sole wear is found in the runner whose foot supinates excessively during running. The supinator's sole wear pattern is the exact opposite of that found in the pronator, as the main wear is concentrated on the outer border of the sole, from heel to toe (shoe below).

The extent that excessive outer sole wear, particularly at the heel, influences injury risk is uncertain. There is indeed some merit in the argument that wear, particularly at the heel, is an adaptation to the individual athlete's particular mechanical make-up. So if an athlete's shoes wear rapidly at the heel, they have a reason for doing so. This argument suggests that regularly re-patching the heel may be wrong and may be a factor in injury. Experiment cautiously here to establish whether repairing the outer-sole either increases or reduces the liklihood of injury for you.

Stretching

Training promotes muscle strength and flexibility imbalances. Every kilometre we run increases the strength and inflexibility of the muscles most active in endurance running — the posterior calf, hamstring and back muscles — with a corresponding reduction of strength in their opposing muscles, the front calf, front thigh and stomach muscles. The strength and flexibility imbalances may ultimately become an important factor in injury and many authorities (but not all) believe that it is important to maintain flexibility by stretching regularly.

Stretching is not something that most runners do willingly. Runners who will somehow squeeze in one or two hours of running a day, never seem quite able to find the additional five to ten minutes needed for adequate stretching. There are a variety of reasons for this.

Firstly, we inflexible runners are unconvinced that stretching is beneficial; secondly, we are ignorant of what is involved;

Colleen de Reuck

(see page 33)

Interview

I developed plantar fasciitis in January 1994 when training for the Boston Marathon. Fortunately, by using massage and ice techniques, I was able to train through the injury. I tried to wear orthotics, which cost me $400, but they were not really effective.

What helped me was a muscle balance treatment through the use of 'yellow pages' fitted into my shoe as a wedge support. After that was done, my injury cleared up almost immediately.

Our comment

'Yellow pages' is an unconventional treatment, meaning precisely what the name implies. Practitioners of this treatment cut shoe-shaped wedges of yellow pages from telephone directories and insert them into the running shoe of the injured or injury-prone runner.

A sceptical scientist would be forgiven if he or she were to point out that, despite their widespread use and clear effectiveness in aiding recovery from many running injuries, the scientific value of 'yellow pages' is yet to be proven. The same applies to the use of orthotics.

Elana Meyer, Zola Pieterse and members of the winning SA team in the 1995 Rugby World Cup are other elite athletes who have benefited from the 'yellow pages' treatment.

---

thirdly, experience has taught us that stretching hurts; and finally, we are haunted by the suspicion that we may be doing it wrong anyway. None of these is a good enough reason!

The benefits of stretching

Three main benefits have been attributed to regular stretching: these are a reduced risk of injury, less muscle soreness after exercise, and improved athletic performance.

It appears that after a strenuous run athletes are most stiff in the muscles that were least supple before the run. It is also apparent that tightness in certain muscle groups can affect speed. For instance, an athlete's ability to run fast downhill could be limited because of excessive tightness in both the hamstrings and quadriceps muscle groups. Tightness in either of these muscle groups must limit stride length and therefore speed when running downhill, particularly near the end of the race when fatigue has caused the muscles to become even tighter.

At present there is little evidence to suggest that runners who stretch are less prone to injury, but tight calf muscles tend to exacerbate ankle inflexibility, a possible cause of bone strain. Regular stretching of these muscles could limit the occurrence of this injury and others, such as plantar fasciitis.

Perhaps the greatest benefit of regular stretching is seen in those who frequently experience muscle cramps (page 84) during exercise. We have found that the most successful way of preventing these cramps is to undertake a regular stretching programme of up to ten minutes a day. The programme should focus on the muscles that are most prone to cramping during exercise. We postulate that regular stretching prevents the development of cramps by altering the sensitivity of the stretch reflexes, in particular the inverse stretch reflex.

The dangers of stretching
Some runners may become sore and even injured after stretching, but this is most likely because they do not stretch properly.

The physiology of stretching
Muscles have a complicated mechanism that prevents their ever being damaged by overstretching. Muscles contain tiny 'stretch receptors' which are attached to the working part of the muscle — the muscle fibres. When a muscle is stretched, the degree of stretch is sensed by the stretch receptors. As the intensity of the stretch increases, so the stretch receptors begin to fire more rapidly and more strongly. Ultimately, when these impulses exceed a certain threshold, the stretched muscle contracts and shortens, thereby preventing it being overstretched.

A general rule is that the intensity of the muscle contraction induced by a stretch reflex varies with the rapidity with which the stretch was applied. The faster the stretch is applied, the more powerful the contraction it evokes.

Another important stretch reflex, the inverse stretch reflex, performs an exactly opposite function to that of the conventional stretch reflex. Its receptors are centred not among the muscle fibres, but in the muscle tendons. In contrast to the conventional reflex, when these tension receptors in the inverse stretch reflex are activated they inhibit the contraction of that muscle. Therefore the inverse stretch reflex provides a protective mechanism which prevents a muscle from contracting so strongly that it ruptures itself.

The applied physiology of stretching

The above information indicates that the stretch must be applied gradually. A slow build-up of stretch has the least stimulatory effect on the stretch receptors. Thus these receptors remain unstimulated and the tension build-up in the stretched muscle is kept to a minimum. This is important because research has shown that the most effective stretches are achieved when the tension inside the stretched muscles is low.

Secondly, the inverse stretch reflex explains why a muscle that has gradually stretched for sixty to ninety seconds will suddenly 'give' as the inverse stretch relaxes any remaining tension in the stretched muscle.

Stretching techniques

Ballistic stretching

This is the technique beloved of school coaches and rugby players, the flamboyant bobbing up and down while touching one's toes that looks so impressive. Ballistic stretching can also be done by bobbing on the ball of the foot of a straightened leg thrust out behind the body. The front leg is bent at the knee and the legs are alternated frequently. Unfortunately all that ballistic stretching achieves is to activate the stretch reflex, causing the stretched muscle to contract rapidly and the athlete to bob up.

It is found that the tension inside the muscle during ballistic stretching is about twice that in a static stretch. Thus the risk of injury is increased for those who choose this type of stretching.

Passive stretching

In passive stretching, a partner is used to apply additional external pressure to increase the extent of the stretch. This method is particularly popular amongst gymnasts. While this stretching method can be very valuable for expert stretchers, it is potentially risky for inexperienced stretchers.

Contract–relax stretching

Here the muscle to be stretched is first actively contracted, and then stretched immediately it relaxes. The theory behind this technique is that the active muscle contraction activates the

Antonio Pinto *(Portugal)*

Born in 1966, son of a farmer. Worked on farm and construction sites. Started sporting career as a cyclist but at twenty switched to running as it was a higher profile sport. Won 10 000 m at European Championships in 1991, and national titles at cross-country (1992) and 5000 m (1994). Won 1992 London Marathon (2:10:02), and finished third in 1995 (2:08:48), after leading through 40 km. Set personal bests in 10 000 m (27:48) and the marathon (2:08:31) in 1994, winning the Berlin Marathon in the process. Second Portuguese athlete home (22nd) at 1995 World Cross-Country Championships.

Interview

Apart from an ITB injury which I was able to run through, and a minor foot injury, it has been sickness rather than injury which has troubled me. Bad tooth-ache and sinusitis limited my success at the 1992 Olympics and the 1994 European Championships.

My upbringing on the farm helped me to become physically strong, and I think this has helped to keep me mostly free of injuries. My father's farm was on a steep slope, so I suppose that helped to build stamina as well. I did a lot of physical work until I was in a position to concentrate full time on running. Although I now own a wine farm, others do the work!

I stretch regularly, usually in the middle of training sessions and again at the end, as I believe that flexibility is important .

Our comment

Not all injuries that limit an athlete's training and racing performances are orthopaedic. Pinto's story includes two episodes of chronic infections that developed prior to major championships. Heavy training and competitive stress may reduce the athlete's resistance to infection, increasing the probability that a serious infection will develop. The use of anti-oxidant vitamins (C, E and beta-carotene) may increase the athlete's resistance and should be used by athletes prone to developing infection at times of increased training or competitive stress. Pinto's disciplined stretching regime is an example to all.

---

inverse stretch reflex. Thus it is expected that the muscle tension during the subsequent contraction will be reduced. In fact, it has been found that this does not occur. Rather, the contracted muscle continues to be slightly active during the subsequent stretch. Thus the tension in the stretched muscle is actually higher, not lower, than during a static stretch.

Static stretching
Here the stretch position is assumed slowly and held for at least thirty to sixty seconds. As there is a slow build-up of tension in the muscle the stretch reflex is not activated. As the tendons are gradually stretched, the inverse stretch reflex is activated and muscle tension falls, allowing the muscle to be stretched further. As static stretching causes the least muscle tension build-up, it is believed to be most effective.

Maintaining flexibility
Once the desired degree of flexibility has been achieved, a single stretching session once or twice a week will maintain that flexibility. Continuing to stretch three to five times a week will produce further, albeit small, improvements in flexibility.

Planning a stretching programme
The following are guidelines for successful stretching:
- [ ] Results can only be expected after weeks or months. Thus a stretching programmes should be followed all year round or it should begin at least six weeks before the season starts.
- [ ] It is best to stretch both before and after exercise. If this is not possible, stretch before exercise. Increased muscle flexibility after a period of stretching lasts for up to three hours.
- [ ] A short warm-up jog before stretching can be helpful.
- [ ] Select stretching exercises carefully. Start with the easiest and build up to the more advanced.
- [ ] Alternate the muscles that are stretched.
- [ ] Assume the stretching position slowly and hold it for thirty to sixty seconds. The muscle should be stretched to the point where tightness is felt in it. At no time should the stretch cause discomfort or pain.
- [ ] The stretches particularly useful for runners are shown on the following pages. Exercises 1,2,3,4,7,11 (or 8) and 14 can be used if you do not have enough time for them all.
- [ ] Some exercises commonly used by runners (exercises 16–18) are considered risky for inexperienced stretchers and should be replaced by appropriate stretches from exercises 1–15.
- [ ] Do each of the exercises which follow for both sides of the body.

Some useful stretching exercises
These exercises are demonstrated by Tanya Peckham, one of South Africa's finest middle-distance athletes.

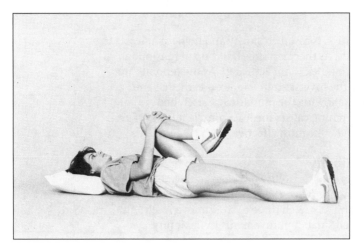

1. Hamstrings
Gradually pull your knee up to your chest. Your head should rest on a comfortable support to enable the neck to relax.

2. Quadriceps
Grasp your foot with your hand as shown and gently pull the foot towards your buttocks. This exercise and exercise 9 should be avoided by athletes who have injured knees as the flexion of the knee joint in these positions may be painful.

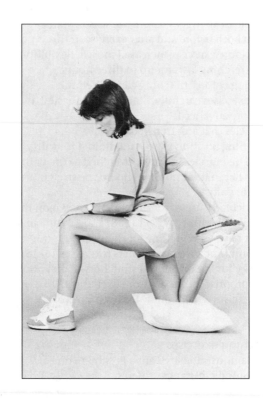

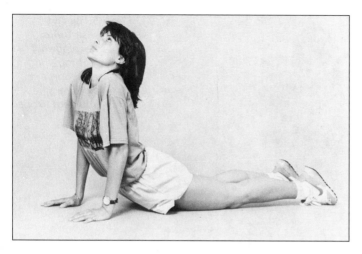

3. Abdomen and chest

Push your upper torso back with your arms. Push your head as far back as it will go.

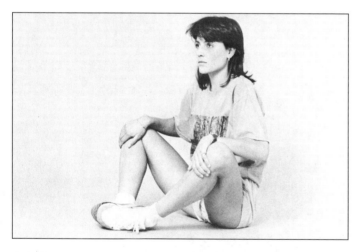

4. Groin

With your back straight and feet together, push down gently on your knees. Alternatively, assume the same position but grasp your toes with your hands. Pull the soles of your feet together, then pull your heels towards your groin as you pull your body forwards.

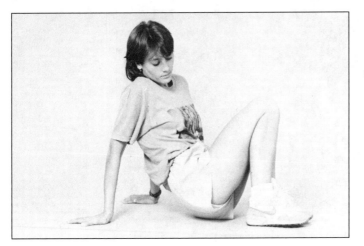

5. Hip and sartorius
Keeping your legs together and your feet stationary, move your legs to one side.

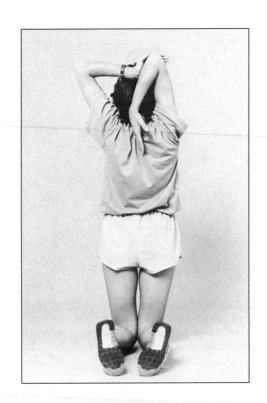

6. Shoulders
Put your elbow behind your head. Then gently pull your elbow towards the centre of your back.

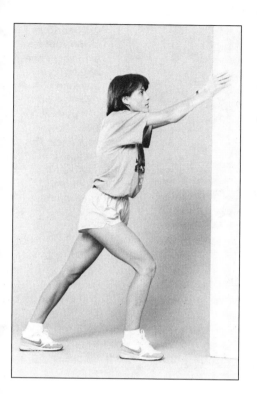

7. Lower leg
Lean against a wall with your back foot flat and your head up. Slowly bend your arms and lower your body towards the wall.

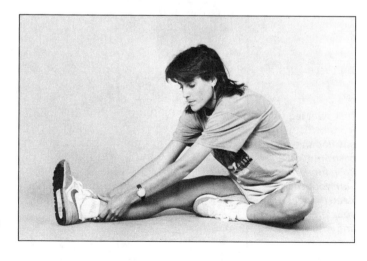

8. Hamstrings
From the position shown, grasp your ankle and pull your body forward. Maintain as straight a back as possible.

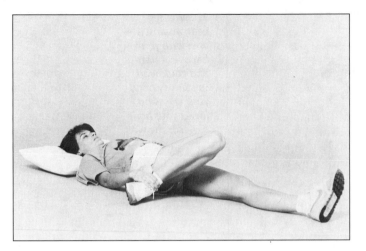

9. Quadriceps
Lie on your back with your knee up and your leg pulled in towards your side as shown. Slowly lower your knee. This exercise is not advised for runners with knee injuries.

10. Lower leg
From the position shown, push your left knee forward with your chest. Keep the toes of your left foot in line with the knee of your right leg.

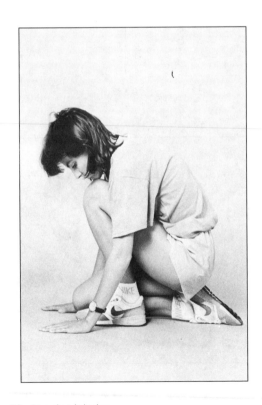

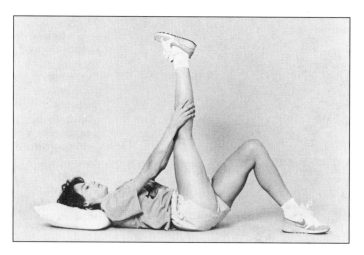

11. Hamstrings

Grasp your leg below the calf and pull it towards your head. This stretch achieves maximum benefit if you use a cord or belt around the arch of your foot to pull the straightened leg towards your head. The head should be supported and the neck as relaxed as possible.

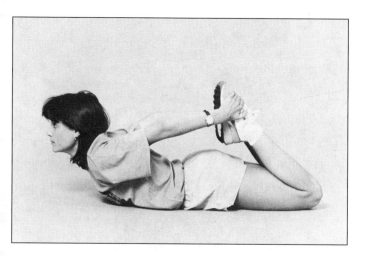

12. Abdomen and chest

Grasp both feet above the ankles. Arch your back and pull your feet towards your head.

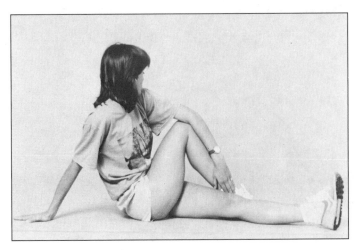

**13. Hip and
sartorius**
*Cross your right
leg over your left
leg and bring
your left arm
through as
shown. Push
against your leg
with your arm,
twisting your
body and
turning your
head towards
the back as you
do so.*

**14. Iliotibial
band**
*Put your weight
on your left leg
and cross your
right leg in front
of it. Bend
towards the
right, pushing
your hips
towards the left
as shown.*

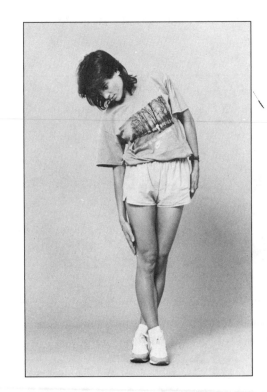

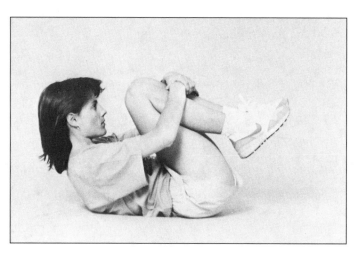

15. Back and hamstrings
Rock gently back and forth eight to ten times. Always do this exercise before exercise 17 because it gently pre-stretches the back muscles.

16. Hamstrings (high risk)
This exercise must be preceded by a warm-up and should be attempted only by experienced stretchers. The force of gravity pulling on the trunk places a heavy load on the spine and lower back muscles, so the exercise could be dangerous for those with lower back problems. Avoid the temptation to 'bounce' while doing this stretch. The movement must be solely through rotation of your hips, the back kept straight. The risk can be reduced by placing your hands on a table in front of you to take some of the weight. This will ease the load on your spine.

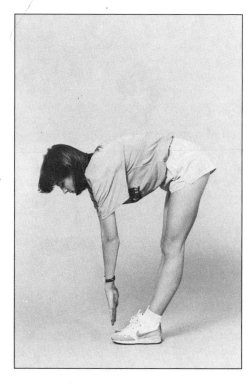

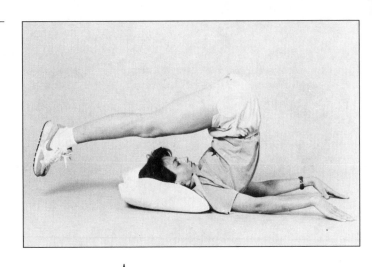

17. Back and hamstrings (high risk)

The exercise above, 'the plough', is for experienced stretchers who have no back problems. The risk can be reduced by supporting your back with your hands, your upper arms maintaining floor balance and your ankles flexed. This prevents you from stretching beyond what your flexibility will allow. Always do exercise 15 before this stretch.

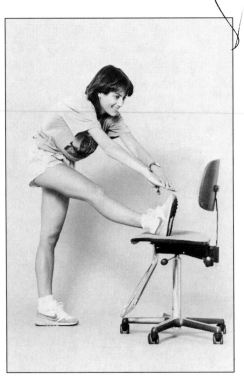

18. Hamstrings (high risk)

This exercise is very popular among runners, who tend simply to walk up to a wall and fling their leg against it. They begin the exercise with the leg extended at ninety degrees and then apply force to stretch it further. However, since the average runner is not flexible enough to cope with this, the risk of injury is high. For experienced runners only.

Use this simple checklist to stay injury-free:

☑ *Run on forgiving surfaces*
Ideal running surfaces are firm, flat (not cambered) and smooth, and should provide some shock absorption. Surfaces in order of most to least desirable: cinder track; artificial track; firm dirt path; grass; tarmac; hard gravel path; concrete.

☑ *Warm up before (and cool down after)*
An adequate warm-up reduces the risk of a muscle or tendon injury during a hard training session. Cooling down may improve recovery from a hard training session or race.

☑ *Stretch regularly*
This maintains the flexibility of the muscles and tendons.

☑ *Alternate hard and easy training days*
This allows the body, especially the muscles, a chance to recover fully from the previous heavy training session. While most runners need to have at least two easy days between hard training sessions, some runners need up to six.

☑ *Race in moderation and only when injury-free*
One rule holds that at least one day's rest (from racing) should be allowed for each kilometre that one races at distances up to 15 km. For longer distances the rest period between races should be much longer. Run marathons as infrequently as one every six months; and longer races only once every year.

☑ *Maintain a daily running logbook*
The logbook allows one to distinguish, in retrospect, between programmes that produced success and those that were less effective. An accurate record of training volume also indicates how much training the athlete can sustain without injury, or conversely, the amount of training that is likely to produce injury.

☑ *Monitor your running shoes*
Keep a regular check on your shoes to ensure that they have not worn excessively and that the mid-soles have not compacted, as discussed on page 40.

5 The ten laws of running injuries

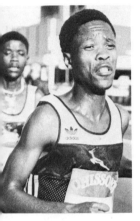

Unique features of running injuries

It is absolutely crucial to understand the reason for a running injury. It serves no purpose to diagnose the injury correctly if no attention is paid to the cause. If nothing is done to eliminate the gremlin that caused the injury to appear in the first place, the injury is quite likely to recur, possibly more seriously than before. This chapter is intended to allow you to reflect on why your injury occurred. This reflection will ensure that you continue to enjoy running for years to come instead of ending your career on the runners' scrapheap. To this end we print here an edited and updated version of Noakes's Ten Laws of Running Injuries, adapted from *Lore of Running*.

The first law of running injuries

Running injuries are not an act of God. They result from the interaction of the athlete's genetic structure with the environment, through training methods

As already described on page 8, running injuries are not extrinsic injuries as contact sport injuries are. They are intrinsic injuries resulting from the interaction of the athlete's training methods, training environment and genetic structure. In other words, running injuries happen for a reason and this reason can be discovered through examining the three factors mentioned above.

The second law of running injuries

Each running injury progresses through four stages or grades
Unlike extrinsic injuries, in which the onset is almost always sudden and dramatic — such as the rugby player being caught in a ferocious tackle — the onset of intrinsic running-related injury is almost always gradual. Running injuries become gradually and progressively more debilitating, typically passing through four stages or grades.

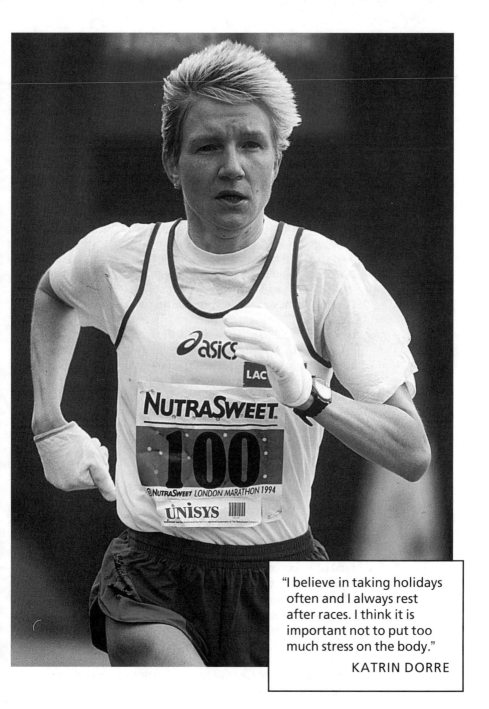

"I believe in taking holidays often and I always rest after races. I think it is important not to put too much stress on the body."

KATRIN DORRE

A grade I running injury is one that causes pain only after exercise and is often felt only some hours afterwards. A grade II injury is one that causes discomfort, not yet pain, during exercise, but which is insufficiently severe to reduce the athlete's training or racing performance. A grade III injury, on the other hand, causes more severe discomfort, now recognized as pain, that limits the athlete's training and interferes with racing performance. Finally, a grade IV injury is so severe that it prevents any attempts at running.

Grading injuries in this way allows a more rational approach to treatment. An athlete with a grade I injury requires less active treatment than the athlete with a grade IV injury. Similarly, the athlete with a grade I injury does not have to be excessively concerned as long as the injury does not progress to grade II. If it does so, it will need more serious attention.

Secondly, you need not fear that a grade I injury you have had for some time will suddenly deteriorate overnight into a grade IV injury. (The only exceptions to this rule are stress fractures and the iliotibial band friction syndrome, both of which can become incapacitatingly severe with alarming rapidity).

Thirdly, the grade of the injury helps the doctor define each athlete's pain or anxiety threshold. The athlete who seeks attention for an injury only when it reaches grade IV, clearly has a different anxiety threshold from the athlete who seeks urgent attention for a grade I injury. Obviously the advice given for each type will also differ greatly: the former requires very little psychological support, the latter much more.

The third law of running injuries

Each running injury indicates that the athlete has reached breakdown point

It seems almost certain that every athlete has a potential breakdown point — a training intensity and a racing frequency at which breakdown becomes inevitable. This may be a weekly total of 30 km or 300 km in training or a racing frequency of one or fifty races a year. This law is really a corollary to the first law which holds that there is a reason why running injuries occur. This law simply emphasizes that once an injury has occurred it is time to analyse why the injury has happened at all. This will frequently be because the athlete has reached breakdown point, usually because of some change in training routine. He or she may be training harder or running further, or running on a different terrain or in different or worn-out running shoes.

Katrin Dorre *(Germany)*

One of the world's most consistent marathoners over the past decade, and regarded as the most reliable female marathoner in athletics history. Has bettered 2:30 on no fewer than twelve occasions. Winner of eighteen marathons. Ran PB at Berlin in 1994 (2:25:15) at her 30th attempt at the marathon. The first runner, male or female, to have won the London Marathon three times in succession, having recorded straight victories between 1992 and 1994, with a fastest time of 2:27:09 in 1993. Olympic bronze medal in 1988.

Interview

I think that part of the reason why I've remained injury-free for so long is the fact that running is not the most important thing in my life. My family is. Although I train and race hard (up to 190 miles per week in training, often at altitude), I am not, perhaps, as consumed by running as others are. It is important for me to enjoy the freedom of running because I want to.

Typically, after a marathon, I will take a holiday, and with it a complete break from training. Then I will cross train for two to three months, just swimming and cycling, no running. Then I give myself two to three months to prepare for my next marathon. I think that it is important not to put too much pressure on your body.

I also think that having my daughter, Katharina, in 1988 was good for me. At first I thought that I would have to retire, as in East Germany we were not permitted to go into training camps with our children. But then the wall came down and these restrictions were lifted. So I thought I would make a new beginning. I think starting afresh was good for me. Pregnancy enabled my body to regenerate and take on a new lease of life.

Our comment

Dorre's story is a refreshing challenge to the belief that success in marathon running comes solely as a result of slavish dedication to a single, narrow goal. Many of the really great female distance runners have shown this balance, although it is not easily achieved. Dorre's story suggests that her victories in eighteen marathons, her freedom from injury and her annual break from running training for up to three months — an approach most world-class athletes would consider highly unusual — are probably causally related. Perhaps more runners, especially those prone to chronic or recurrent injuries, might benefit from the Dorre approach.

Alternatively, we are beginning to appreciate that many injuries result simply from continued heavy training over many months. It is remarkable how busy sports doctors become in the months immediately before major events!

The key in the prevention and treatment of injuries is to understand that just as most of us will never win a major race because of certain genetic limitations, so our genes limit our choice of shoes, influence what surfaces we can safely train on, and ultimately determine what training methods we can survive. Only when we learn this perspective will we have sufficient wisdom to be injury resistant. The corollary, of course, is that athletes who are frequently injured are not yet wise enough to appreciate these points. The implication is that when a running injury occurs, the factors that the wise runner needs to consider are the following: training surfaces, training shoes and training methods. These aspects are discussed in detail from page 28 onwards.

The fourth law of running injuries

Virtually all true running injuries are entirely curable

Only a minute fraction of true running injuries are not entirely curable by quite simple techniques and surgery is required in only very exceptional cases. So the injured runner should be reassured that a cure is almost certain. The only possible exceptions to this rule are injuries that:

☐ occur in runners with very severe biomechanical abnormalities for which conventional measures are unable to compensate adequately. However, only a small number of runners have such severe mechanical abnormalities that they are unable to run without injury;
☐ result in severe degeneration of the internal structure of important tissues, in particular the achilles tendon;
☐ occur in those who start running on abnormal joints, in particular hips, knees and ankles;
☐ occur in those with such weak bones that they are forever afflicted by bone injuries such as tibial or fibular bone strain ('shinsplints') or stress fractures.

An important corollary to the fourth law of running injuries is that if you are not completely cured of your running injury by the experts whom you initially consulted, it is time to look elsewhere. But treat even the advice of runners with some caution and do not accept it unconditionally.

The fifth law of running injuries

X-rays and other sophisticated investigations are seldom necessary in the diagnosis of running injuries
Most running injuries affect the soft tissue structures (tendons, ligaments and muscles), particularly those near the major joints. These structures do not show on X-rays: thus one should be wary of the practitioner whose first reaction to your injury is to order an X-ray. Unless that X-ray can be justified, you are probably better off putting the money that would have been spent on the radiological examination, into a good pair of running shoes or other form of preventive treatment, such as this book!

However, new technologies including ultrasound and magnetic resonance image (MRI) scanning are now able to picture the soft tissues. These techniques are extremely useful in diagnosing the true nature of injuries that are resistant to treatment and that are often caused by uncommon or rare conditions.

Bone scanning, in which a radio-labelled tracer is injected into the bloodstream, is also a useful technique for identifying unusual stress fractures (see diagnosis of stress fractures on page 70). The radio-labelled tracer accumulates at the site of bone damage, where the metabolism of the bone cells is most active. When pictured with a special camera, the site of stress fracture shows up as a 'hot spot' in the bone where the radio-labelled tracer has accumulated.

Generally, though, the diagnosis of most running injuries is made with the hands, so the practitioner who does not feel the injured site carefully with his or her hands must always be suspect.

The sixth law of running injuries

Treat the cause, not the effect, of injury
Because all running injuries have a cause, it follows that the injury can never be cured until the causative factors are eliminated. Therefore surgery, physiotherapy, cortisone injections, drug therapy, chiropractic manipulations and homeopathic remedies are likely to fail if they do not correct all the genetic, environmental and training factors causing the runner's injury. It is wise to remember the following axiom: the runner is an innocent victim of a biomechanical abnormality arising in the lower limb. First treat the biomechanical abnormality and then only the injury.

Unfortunately, there are some runners whose injuries exist more in their heads than in their legs. These athletes are characterized by their failure to respond to the forms of treatment that would normally be expected to succeed.

The seventh law of running injuries

Rest is seldom the most appropriate treatment

If an injury is caused solely by running, then the logical answer for those who know no better is to advise avoidance of running (rest) as the obvious cure. Rest does indeed cure the acute symptoms, but like any therapy that does not aim to correct the cause of the injury, it must ultimately fail in the long term. The reason for this is that as soon as the athlete stops resting and starts running again, the lower limbs are exposed to the same stresses as before, and the injury must inevitably recur.

The only injuries which require complete rest are usually those which, in any case, make running impossible. For example, athletes with stress fractures simply cannot run however much they may wish to.

A possible approach is to advise runners to continue running, but only to the point where they experience discomfort. They may not run so far that their injury becomes frankly painful.

If the treatment is effective, then the runner's discomfort should become progressively less during running, making it possible to run progressively further.

On the other hand, if the pain does not improve on treatment, then either the treatment is ineffective or else the diagnosis is wrong.

Furthermore, if the injury does not respond to what should be adequate treatment within three to five weeks, then the alarm bells must ring very, very loudly. The failure of an injury to respond indicates that it might be an obscure injury such as effort thrombosis of the deep veins in the calf. It may also be an injury unrelated to running, for example a bone cancer for which another form of treatment may be urgently required.

The eighth law of running injuries

Never accept, as a final opinion, the advice of a non-runner (medical doctor or other)

There are strong grounds for believing that everyone considers themselves an expert on sport. People who are otherwise extremely wary about expressing opinions on subjects about which they may actually know something, feel no such restraint when the topic of sport arises. This applies as much to members of the health professions as it does to anyone else.

How, then, do you know whose advice you can trust? There are four simple criteria.

☐ Firstly, your adviser must be either a runner or someone who has made a special study of runners. Without the first hand experience of running, he or she won't have sufficient insight to help you. Of course, this doesn't mean that all the advice you get from runners will be sound — only that there is a greater probability that it will be correct.

☐ Secondly, your adviser must be able to discuss in detail the genetic, environmental and training factors likely to have caused your injury. If the person you consult is unable to do this, together you will go nowhere.

☐ Thirdly, an adviser who is unable to cure your injury should be hurt by it as much as you are. Your adviser must understand the importance of your running to you. It is patently ridiculous to accept advice from someone who is antagonistic to your running.

☐ Fourthly, your adviser shouldn't be expensive.

The ninth law of running injuries

Avoid the knife

The only running injuries for which surgery is the first line of treatment are muscle compartment syndromes (page 131) and interdigital neuromas (page 160). Surgery may also have a role in the treatment of chronic achilles tendonitis of six or more months duration, low back pain owing to a prolapsed disc and the iliotibial band friction syndrome — but only when all other forms of non-operative treatment have been trialed.

The obvious danger of surgery is that it is irreversible: what is removed at surgery cannot be put back. It is a tragedy, as has happened on more than one occasion, for a runner to have undergone major knee, ankle or back surgery for the wrong diagnosis. Not only will that surgery fail to cure the injury, but it may seriously affect the unfortunate athlete's future career.

Remember that surgery should only be considered for a small group of injuries and only when such injuries are at grade III or, more usually, grade IV, level.

The tenth law of running injuries

There is, as yet, no scientific evidence that running causes (osteo) arthritis in runners whose knees were normal when they started running

Osteoarthritis is a degenerative disease in which the articular cartilage lining the bony surfaces inside the knee joint becomes progressively thinner. Eventually the bone beneath the cartilage on both sides of the joints (usually the hips or knees in runners) becomes exposed. In the advanced stages of osteoarthritis the exposed bones rub against each other, causing pain and severely limited joint movement. The view of some medical professionals is that this degenerative process can be initiated and exacerbated by long-distance running.

However, the entire scientific literature does not contain one scrap of published evidence suggesting that running can initiate the development of osteoarthritis in people who begin running with normal joints. In fact, what evidence there is presents an entirely different picture. Notes on some of these scientific studies can be found in *Lore of Running*.

Sportspeople who develop osteoarthritis have usually had joint surgery and have exercised on these abnormal joints.

The type of sports injury that requires surgery is the one resulting from the typical extrinsic injuries that occur in contact sports. So those who blame running as a cause of osteoarthritis are barking up the wrong tree. Banning contact sports would do more to prevent osteoarthritis in the community than banning running would!

In conclusion   In summarizing these ten laws it seems that in many ways the medical approach to running injuries is the medicine of a bygone era. A correct diagnosis requires a careful, unhurried approach in which the patient is given sufficient time to detail the full story and recount training methods. The doctor must have the time and patience to listen carefully and sympathetically. Seldom is it necessary to utilize expensive tests to establish the diagnosis, and the treatment prescribed is usually very simple. Indeed, it is possible that sixty percent of the doctor's success is due to an ability to understand what the injury means to the patient, the fears that the injury engenders and how best to allay those fears. For this the doctor needs to understand the patient's psyche and understand why the patient came to have the injury examined.

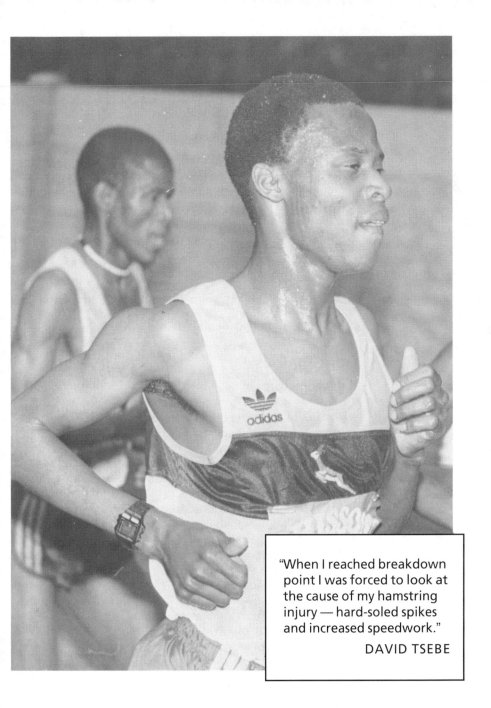

"When I reached breakdown point I was forced to look at the cause of my hamstring injury — hard-soled spikes and increased speedwork."

DAVID TSEBE

6 Bones and muscles

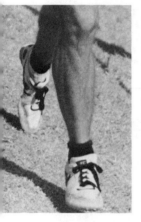

A discussion of non-site-specific injuries

Similar injuries at different sites

This chapter contains a general account of certain types of bone and muscle injuries which occur at different sites on the musculo-skeletal system. While the site of injury may vary, the diagnosis, cause and treatment are frequently the same. This chapter provides a background to the discussion of site-specific injuries in the last chapter, and cross-references are therefore made between the two for ease of comparison.

Bone injuries

Stress fractures

Unlike the common bone fractures occurring in contact sports like rugby, in which a single external blow causes the bone to fracture, the runner's bone may fracture as a result of repetitive minor trauma accumulating over weeks or months.

It is a concept that runners usually find difficult to accept. How can something as strong as bone fracture so easily, they want to know?

The answer is that bone injuries occur in runners whose bones are too weak (for reasons detailed below) to cope with the load to which they are exposed in running.

The diagram on page 70 indicates the tibia (large shin bone) to be the most vulnerable to stress fractures. The tibia is followed, in order of frequency of occurrence, by the metatarsals (toe bones), the fibula (small calf bone), the femur (thigh bone), the navicular (ankle bone) and the pubic bone (groin).

The pain associated with a stress fracture is usually bearable when at rest or when walking, but as soon as any running is attempted, it becomes quite unbearable and running is impossible.

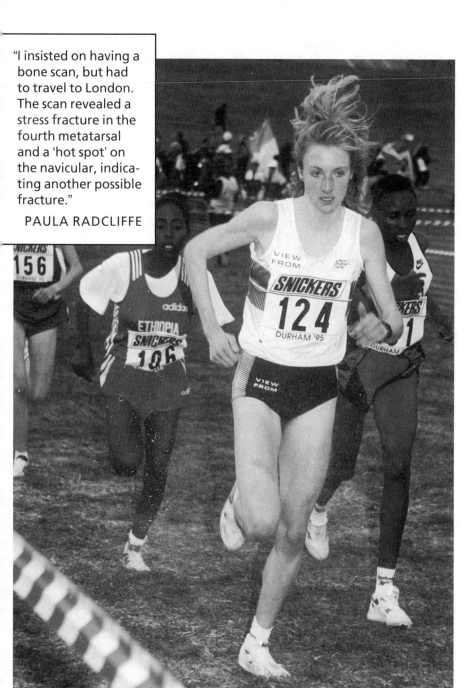

> "I insisted on having a bone scan, but had to travel to London. The scan revealed a stress fracture in the fourth metatarsal and a 'hot spot' on the navicular, indicating another possible fracture."
>
> PAULA RADCLIFFE

Diagnosis

The diagnosis of a stress fracture is quite simple:

- ☐ The injury is usually of quite sudden onset and there is no history of external violence. Runners get little notice of the tragedy about to befall them. Then suddenly they are no longer able to run. An injury that prevents running is almost always a stress fracture.
- ☐ The runner will find that standing on one leg may be painful, if not impossible (fracture of the pelvis). Alternatively, hopping on the injured leg is almost always painful in the other fractures.
- ☐ Extreme tenderness, localized to the bone, is felt when the injured site is pressed.
- ☐ The injury heals itself completely within three months of complete rest.

A diagram showing the percentage of stress fractures occurring at different sites of the anatomy

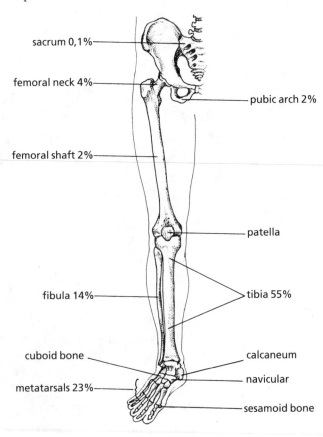

sacrum 0,1%

femoral neck 4%

pubic arch 2%

femoral shaft 2%

patella

fibula 14%

tibia 55%

cuboid bone

calcaneum

navicular

metatarsals 23%

sesamoid bone

A general rule for the rate of healing is that the further the site is from the centre of gravity of the body, the shorter the healing period. Thus stress fractures of the foot can heal within five weeks, whereas those of the pelvis can take up to five months before recovery is complete.

Unfortunately, few runners will accept a lengthy rest period without some visible evidence that the diagnosis is correct. So we usually have to resort to X-rays and bone scans, both of which are not without their own drawbacks. X-rays will often fail to reveal the presence of a stress fracture if they are taken earlier than three weeks after the initial injury. In effect, the fracture is so small that it cannot be seen. Only when new bone is being formed, which is more dense than the old bone it replaces, does the fracture show as a line on the X-ray.

A technique which can be used to detect stress fractures is 'bone scanning', which indicates as 'hotspots' areas of high bone cell activity, such as at the site of a fracture. It can be argued, however, that bone scanning for these injuries is really only necessary either if the injury fails to heal within six weeks (for smaller bones) to twelve weeks (for larger bones such as the femur, tibia and pelvis) or if it recurs within a few weeks of the runner starting to run again. Neither of these are features of a conventional stress fracture and would indicate the need for a thorough evaluation to exclude another cause of pain, such as bone cancer, unrelated to running.

Cause

The exact reason why stress fractures occur is not known, but there appears to be an abnormal concentration of stress at a particular site in the bone which is insufficiently strong at that site to resist those forces. It is now clear that the initial response in bones subjected to increased loading is the activation of specialized cells, osteoclasts, whose function it is to cause bone resorption. During this process, bone cells are absorbed back by the body. This process is known as 'osteoclonal excavation'. During this phase bone strength is likely to be reduced, placing the bone at increased risk of fracture.

This process of bone resorption passes gradually into a phase in which new bone is laid down by other specialized bone cells, the osteoblasts. Stress fractures (and bone strain) develop in those whose bones either undergo excessive osteoclonal excavation or whose osteoblastic response is either delayed or initially ineffectual.

Frith van der Merwe *(South Africa)*

Best ultra-distance athlete in the world in the history of women's competition. Performances in the 1989 Comrades and Two Oceans Marathons surpass all other female ultra-distance efforts. Set world 30 mile (3:01:16) and 50 km (3:08:13) records in completing the Two Oceans 56 km race (which includes two severe hill climbs) in 3:30:36. These records still stood in 1995, and were considerably quicker than the world track equivalents of 3:19:41 and 3:26:45 held by Carolyn Hunter-Rowe. Her 50 mile time of 5:20 (no official time recorded) in the 88 km Comrades Marathon in 1980 is twenty minutes faster than American Ann Trason's official world best of 5:40:18.

Won national titles over 15 km in 1989 (49:44) and the marathon in 1990 (2:27:36). Half-marathon and 10 km bests of 1:11:42 and 33:19. Won 1991 Comrades in 6:08. Injured in first half of 1992 but ran 2:39:24 at Berlin Marathon. Placed seventh in 2:35:56 at World Championships in Stuttgart in 1993. Attempted comeback at Comrades in 1994 but forced out after 30 km with stress fracture.

As Frith Agliotti, won several road races in 1995, including a course record of 2:46:55 at altitude in the Elands Valley Marathon.

Interview   *My stress fracture [of the heel bone] came as an enormous shock to me — I think it was one of the biggest blows in my life. Everyone had been warning me that I'd become injured because of my heavy racing schedule, but of course I never believed them! And then it happened, at the worst possible time.*

The injury forced me to rest and reflect on why it had happened. I realized that it was entirely my fault and that there had been a reason for the injury. For one thing, I had been racing far too much. I discovered another when I was found to have very low oestrogen levels and I was also low on calcium.

I began to think more positively and bought myself an exercise bike, which I worked out on twice a day. At first the injury was very painful and I couldn't even walk down stairs, but I forced myself to be patient. I slept with an 'electrical bandage' around my ankle, which subjected the bone to an electrical field. This speeded recovery.

In retrospect I'm not sorry it happened to me, and I believe I will be a better runner for it. I had been abusing my body, not listening to what it was telling me. I'd race an ultra-marathon one day and be out training the next.

Our comment   Frith's running career has been characterized by a three year period of exceptional performances in which she ran world-class times at distances from 15 km to 90 km, and a longer period in which she became injured and has not run as fast again. Her experience, and that of other marathon and ultra-marathon runners in both South Africa and overseas, seems to indicate that the human body can produce only a very limited number of exceptional marathon and ultra-marathon races. These must be carefully planned and cherished. Greed is a natural enemy to success. A relatively minor injury like a stress fracture may be the first sign of the threat that greed can become.

The real tragedy, which the athlete may only appreciate too late, is that once the body has been, in Frith's term, 'abused', there may never be a full recovery.

Nutrition seems to play an important role in maintaining long-term performance. Empirical observation suggests that runners who continue eating healthily without restricting the energy contents of their diets may survive for longer at the top. In contrast, those athletes who actively reduce their energy intake in order to be thinner in the belief that they will run faster may soon discover that this approach works only in the short term. The challenge, especially for female athletes, is to resist the pressure to achieve a body-fat content as close to zero as possible.

Muscles, not fat, propel the human body; the extreme diets needed to achieve zero percent body fat also reduce muscle mass and therefore reduce the size of the very engine that is needed to achieve excellence.

The concept of sustainability merits consideration in athletics, where greatness is usually measured simply in terms of times or distance. But are not the truly great athletes those who consistently produce top performances? This would set athletes such as Katrin Dorre (see page 61) and Bruce Fordyce (see page 17) apart from the Chinese one-year-wonder Wang Junxia, despite her spectacular performances.

Various risk factors for stress fractures have been identified:

Female sex
Women are more prone to stress fractures than men. It has been shown that the frequency of stress fractures in women is up to twelve times higher than in men. Women who experience menstrual abnormalities are especially at risk.

Training errors

Most stress fractures occur in novice runners — or in competitive runners who suddenly increase their training load, run one or more very long races, return too quickly to heavy training or sustain a very heavy training and racing programme for many months. Hard training during the early period of bone weakening is more likely to cause a fracture. Novice runners are particularly vulnerable eight to twelve weeks after training begins, for it is then that their increased muscle and heart fitness allows them to train much harder at the exact time when their bones are not yet strong enough to cope with the added stress of heavier training.

Another adverse feature of suddenly increasing one's training distance is that it causes accumulated muscular fatigue which may then reduce the muscles' ability to absorb shock — a function which is then passed on to the bones, which are thus more likely to fracture. Also see page 30.

Shoes

Excessively hard running shoes, in particular training spikes in track athletes or shoes with compacted EVA, may be a factor explaining this injury. However, it seems that shoes play less of a role in this injury than do major errors in training methods.

Genetic factors

Three principal genetic factors are associated with stress fractures — the high-arched foot which fails to absorb shock adequately and is associated with fractures of the femur (thigh bone) and metatarsals (toe bones); the pronating low-arched foot which causes abnormal biomechanical function in the lower limb, predisposing the tibia (large calf bone) and the fibula (small calf bone) to fractures; and leg-length inequalities.

Menstrual abnormalities or a low-calcium diet or both

There is growing evidence that the bones of the majority of female sportspeople who have abnormal menstrual patterns are likely to become weaker. This happens firstly because the blood levels of the female hormone oestrogen, which is required for normal bone mineralization, are depressed and secondly because their dietary calcium intake may be too low to maintain normal bone mineral content. Their weaker bones are more prone to bone strain injuries and stress fractures.

Studies have shown that the dietary calcium intakes of

sportspeople with shin soreness (stress fractures or tibial or fibular bone strain) is abnormally low and could be a predisposing factor for the injury. Alternatively, it may be that the diets of these injured runners are inadequate in everything — calories, protein and minerals — not only calcium.

Treatment

The only treatment required for most stress fractures is six to twelve weeks' rest. Because these fractures seldom become unstable and therefore liable to go out of alignment, they do not need to be placed in plaster of Paris. This treatment can actually cause muscle weakening and bone demineralization. Some form of bandaging may reduce discomfort in the early weeks following injury.

More recently, three methods have been proposed for possibly shortening the healing process. These are:

☐ exposing the fracture to an electrical field;
☐ exercising in water in a specially designed pool using a flotation device;
☐ exposing the fracture to an increased pressure in a compression (hyperbaric) chamber.

Further research is required before the effectiveness of these methods is known. One more cynical view of the value of hyperbaric therapy for bone fractures — a form of treatment to which the fractured hand of star South African fullback Andre Joubert was subjected during the 1995 Rugby World Cup — is that it is 'a therapy in search of a disease'! But the same could be said of many forms of treatment that are routinely prescribed for the management of sports injuries. Many have become popular before they have been subjected to rigorous clinical trials to determine their real benefits.

Alternatively, runners with fractures of the tibia or fibula may achieve complete relief from their symptoms and may be able to continue their activities by wearing a pneumatic leg brace.

There is one exception to the general rule that stress fractures do not need to be immobilized. A stress fracture of the neck of the femur is an extremely serious injury and, as the injury can have dire consequences, requires the urgent attention of an orthopaedic surgeon.

But the real challenge for runners recovering from all stress fractures other than that of the femoral neck, is to keep

Paula Radcliffe *(United Kingdom)*

Started running aged five when she accompanied her mother and brother while seconding her father on his long training runs. Insisted on jogging a few kilometres on these occasions. She placed 299th in the under thirteen age group in her national cross-country championships, training just one day a week. Then gave up judo sessions and trained twice a week to finish fourth in the same division the following year in 1987! Progressed in cross-country and won the British under seventeen title in 1991. Won British junior title in 1992 and a month later won the World Junior (under twenty) Cross-Country title at Boston. Ran for Britain at the World Junior Track Championships in Seoul in 1992, where she placed fourth in the 3000 m in 8:51 and at the Senior Championships in Stuttgart in 1993, where she placed seventh in the 3000 m final in a PB of 8:40:40. Placed fifth in the 5000 m at the 1995 World Track Championships at Göteborg, Sweden, in a PB of 14:57. She finished 18th at senior level at the World Cross-Country Championships in 1993 (Amorebieta, Spain) and again in 1995 (Durham, UK), shortly after an injury-enforced lay-off, after dropping off the lead pack in the final kilometre.

Interview

I'd had a solid 1993 season and started 1994 well, with wins in World Cross Challenge [cross-country] races in Durham and Belfast. I won the national trials race in February, but my foot started hurting afterwards. I won the national cross-country championships in March, but the pain in my foot had worsened and it hurt to raise my toes.

A physiotherapist diagnosed strained tendons and then a dropped arch, and prescribed orthotics. I ran 400 m on the track with the orthotic and stopped. I couldn't even walk and I was forced to withdraw from the World Cross-Country Championships. Still the physiotherapist did not believe it to be a fracture and I had some ultrasound treatment. I was unable to have a bone scan, but an MRI scan did not show a stress fracture. The verdict was ligament damage.

I insisted on having a bone scan, but had to travel to London. The scan revealed a stress fracture of the fourth metatarsal and a 'hot spot' on the navicular, indicating another possible fracture.

I spent three weeks in plaster below the knee and concentrated on exercising my upper body and cycling with the cast. Once out of the plaster I spent three more weeks running in a pool and having more physiotherapy, including manipulations.

No one has yet been able to pin-point the cause of the stress fracture. In hindsight, it was a mistake to have my leg in plaster as I lost a lot of muscle, particularly in my calf.

physically active so that they avoid runner's withdrawal symptoms, and to find out why the injury happened in the first place to prevent being thwarted again.

Since dietary calcium intake is low in runners with bone injuries, it makes sense that runners with bone injuries should increase their calcium intakes. But as yet there is no firm evidence that this will reduce the risk of a recurrent injury.

It is generally advisable that women with menstrual disturbances should consult a specialist for advice about the need to take hormone replacement therapy if their menstrual periods do not return with a reduction in training and an increase in dietary energy intake, where appropriate.

Tibial and fibular bone strain ('shinsplints')
As this injury is site-specific to just three localities on the tibia and fibula, it is fully discussed in the Troubleshooter's Guide.

Muscle injuries
Delayed muscle soreness
This takes the form of that feeling of muscle discomfort that comes on twenty-four to forty-eight hours after unaccustomed or particularly severe exercise.

Diagnosis
The diagnosis is straightforward. Muscle pain which peaks twenty-four to forty-eight hours after exercise is indicative that the muscle has been overstressed. Persistent muscle soreness

Xolile Yawa (South Africa)

Born September 1962. SA's most consistent distance athlete between 1980 and 1995. Product of President Brand Gold Mine's sport programme. SA 10 000 m champion for six years in succession from 1985. Set SA 10 000 m record of 27:39:65 in 1987. Best 5000 m time of 13:30:40. Qualified for the 10 000 m final in 1992 Olympics. Placed 13th in 28:37. SA Half-Marathon titles in 1986, 1987 (in his best ever of 1:00:56) and 1988. Second in 1991 and 1995. National 15 km title in 1989. First South African and 12th overall in 1992 World Half-Marathon Championships in 61:48. Won 1993 Berlin Marathon in 2:10:57. Fourth in 1995 London Marathon (behind Ceron, Moneghetti and Pinto) in his best time of 2:10:22.

Interview

In 1990 I had been struggling with a hamstring injury. After treatment it seemed to improve, so I decided to give the Phalaborwa Half-Marathon a go [June 1990]. I finished sixth but could hardly walk afterwards.

I had to withdraw from the SA Half-Marathon Championships [July 1990]. I went to see a specialist but he was unable to find any muscle knot to indicate that it could have been a tear.

In 1987 I developed pain on the outside of my knee. It was particularly bad when I raced the SA Half-Marathon Championships [which he won] and it was with me for about four months. It was diagnosed as ITB syndrome and fortunately when I changed my shoe sponsor and my shoes my problems were resolved. I have not since had a recurrence of the injury.

Then in 1989 I developed calf pain which forced me to drop out of the SA Half-Marathon Championships after just 3 km. Basically I just took a month's break, obtained a new pair of shoes and the injury seemed to heal itself, enabling me to compete in the SA 15 km Championships. [Yawa won the race in a SA record of 43:02, one of the fastest times in the world in 1989.]

Our comment Rest is often one of the best forms of treatment for many running injuries, especially those that heal poorly, like achilles tendonitis or the iliotibial band syndrome. But few elite athletes can take time off from competition or training and so they return to competition before the injury has healed properly. For those not prepared to rest, treatment of acute muscle injuries should include a period of physiotherapy treatment incorporating cross-frictions, stretching, and eccentric muscle strengthening. If the athlete chooses (wisely) also to rest until healed, the same treatment methods should be used. Rest by itself is never an optimum treatment.

The role of shoes in calf muscle injuries is not clear. Perhaps shoes that allow excessive ankle pronation may predispose to calf muscle tears as they did in Bruce Fordyce's case.

The encouraging aspect of Yawa's career is that he has been able to overcome several persistent injuries and has achieved world-class performances over a period of almost fifteen years.

present for days and weeks on end is a strong indicator of overtraining and an absolute indicator of the need to reduce training.

Cause

The likely cause of this delayed muscle soreness is damage of the muscle cells, in particular the connective (supporting) tissue. Recently there have been the very interesting new findings showing that there is frank disruption and death of muscle cells in athletes who complain of pronounced muscle soreness after marathon and ultra-marathon races.

When an unloaded (no force applied) muscle contracts it shortens. This is called a concentric muscular contraction. In contrast, during an eccentric contraction, the muscle length increases when it contracts because the force applied to the muscle exceeds the force produced by the contraction. In running, eccentric muscle contractions occur, especially in the upper thigh (quadriceps) muscles. The force through these muscles becomes very large, particularly as the foot strikes the ground in downhill running.

Repetitive powerful muscle contractions, especially eccentric contractions, cause muscle cell damage by allowing calcium to flood into the cells. This leads to cell death that peaks forty-eight hours after exercise. Initiation of an inflammatory response stimulates nerve endings in the damaged tissue, causing the pain typical of delayed muscle soreness.

Treatment

The only known ways to reduce muscle damage during prolonged exercise are:

- distance training;
- training downhill;
- weight training to increase the strength of the quadriceps muscle. Note that this type of weight training must be done with eccentric contractions.

Interestingly, anti-inflammatory agents appear to have no effect on delayed muscle soreness.

If muscles with delayed soreness are damaged, it would seem logical that rest, with avoidance of further damaging activity, might be the best form of treatment. In fact, new studies suggest that continuing to train vigorously on muscles showing delayed soreness may inhibit recovery.

In conclusion Delayed muscle soreness indicates muscle damage that may have been caused by inappropriate training. The condition may not be as benign as is usually assumed. The best advice at present may be to reduce training substantially or even to rest completely until all traces of muscle discomfort have disappeared.

Chronic muscle tears

Chronic (insidious) muscle tears (muscle knots) are probably the commonest injuries seen in the elite long-distance runners.

The importance of chronic muscle tears is that they are probably the third most common injury among all groups of runners and are especially common among the elite runners; they are usually misdiagnosed, they can be very debilitating and they will respond only to one specific form of treatment.

Diagnosis

- The pain starts gradually, initially coming on after exercise.
- When the pain starts to occur during exercise, it is possible at first to run through the pain. But the pain gets progressively worse until it becomes severe enough to interfere with training. Speedwork, in particular, becomes impossible.
- The pain is almost always localized to a large muscle group, either the buttock, groin, hamstring or calf muscles.
- The pain is deep-seated and can be very severe but passes off rapidly with rest.
- It becomes difficult to push off properly with the toes if the injury is to the calf muscles.
- In contrast to bone injuries, which will improve if sufficient rest is allowed, chronic muscle tears will never improve

unless the correct treatment is prescribed. So the patient can rest for months or even years without any improvement.

☐ To confirm that the injury is indeed a chronic muscle tear, all the runner or, preferably, a physiotherapist or other health professional need do, is to press firmly with two fingers into the affected muscle in the area in which the pain is felt. If it is possible to find a very tender hard 'knot' in the muscle, then the injury is definitely a chronic muscle tear. It is impossible to emphasize sufficiently just how sore these knots are when palpated forcefully — they are excruciating!

Cause

The mechanism of injury in chronic muscle tears is largely unknown. But new evidence suggests that these muscle injuries occur when the muscle is contracting eccentrically. For example, the hamstring muscle is now known to tear when the muscle contracts eccentrically, that is, while it contracts but lengthens during the swing phase of the running cycle, as the muscle contracts to decelerate the foot immediately prior to heel strike (8–11 on pages 51–53).

The calf muscle also tears during the eccentric phase of its contraction, immediately before the heel lifts off the ground as the knee moves forward of the ankle, so stretching the muscle eccentrically (1 and 2 on page 48).

As individuals who have recurrent chronic muscle tears tend to tear the same muscles at the same site every time (usually when they start doing either more speed running or more distance training), it is probable that these tears occur at sites which are exposed to very high loading, typical of fast running.

Because the loading (working against a force) is so concentrated over a small section of the muscle, an initial small tear develops at that site as the muscle gives way. Although the tear is initially too small to cause discomfort, once the initial tear has occurred, a cycle of repair and re-tear develops that leads ultimately to the large tender knot. This probably consists of muscle fibres surrounded by scar tissue.

Experience with our own repetitive and chronic muscle tears, especially in our now-aging muscles, indicates that these muscles tear during eccentric loading. The hamstring tears just before the foot of the affected side hits the ground. The calf muscle tears immediately before the heel lifts off, as the knee moves forward of the ankle, so stretching the calf muscle eccentrically.

It also seems likely that these muscles tear because they do not have sufficient eccentric strength to resist the eccentric loading imposed during the running stride. Evidence for this is still being gathered as it is only recently that specialized machines have been devised to accurately measure eccentric muscle strength. However, it follows that appropriate eccentric muscle strength should be developed in the muscles prone to chronic muscle tears in order to prevent injury.

Treatment

Conventional treatment including drugs and cortisone injections is a waste of time in this injury. The only treatment that works is a physiotherapeutic manoeuvre known as cross-frictions. A better term would be 'crucifixions' because nothing, not even your toughest-ever race, is as painful as cross-frictions applied, however gently, to a chronic muscle tear!

The key to the treatment of these injuries is that a chronic muscle tear will heal only if the cross-frictions are applied to the injury site — the tender knot in the muscle — and if they are applied sufficiently vigorously. If the cross-friction treatment does not reduce the injured athlete to tears, either the diagnosis is wrong, or the physiotherapist is being too kind.

Most chronic muscle tears respond rapidly to a few sessions of cross-frictions. The application of ultrasound treatment immediately following the cross-frictions may be of benefit. The treatment is correct if the pain while running becomes gradually less so that progressively greater distances can be covered at a faster pace. Most injuries will require between five and ten sessions of therapy, each lasting five to ten minutes, after which most runners should be able to run entirely free of pain. Injuries that have lasted for six months or more, may require a longer period of treatment.

As these injuries occur during eccentric contractions, it seems probable that strengthening the affected muscles eccentrically would reduce the risk of re-injury. Walking and running down-hill backwards is a good way to load the calf muscles eccentrically. Eccentric loading of the hamstrings can best be achieved by specific exercises in the gym. These exercises must recreate the action of stopping the foot suddenly as the knee extends.

Because these injuries tend to recur, one should be fastidious about stretching the muscles that tend to be injured. This is especially important before any fast running, in particular before early morning races. Furthermore, it is essential that at

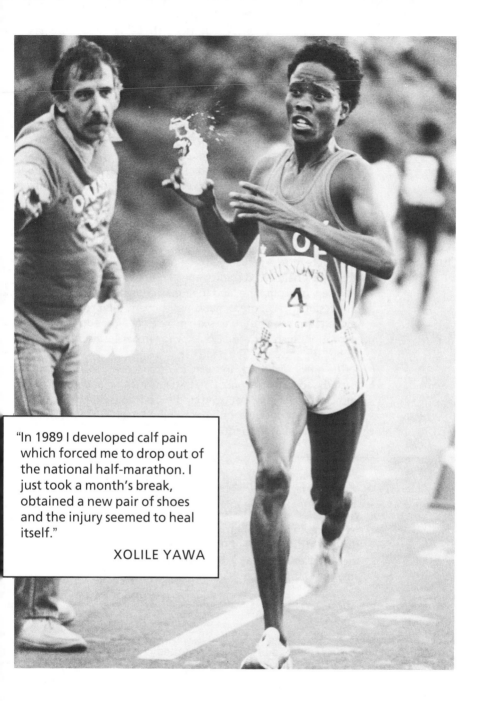

"In 1989 I developed calf pain which forced me to drop out of the national half-marathon. I just took a month's break, obtained a new pair of shoes and the injury seemed to heal itself."

XOLILE YAWA

Elana Meyer (see page 25)

(see page 25)

Interview   *After my first marathon at Boston in 1994, I took several months to recover from the effects of the race. The following year I took a more proactive approach and after the 1995 Boston Marathon went to Florida for ten days to be with a physiotherapist who specializes in recovery techniques.*

Apart from specific muscle massages and stretching exercises, I used the hot and cold bath regime. This involved sitting in an ice bath for fifteen minutes four to five times each day. It was painful, but must have helped as after three or four weeks I felt fully recovered from the effects of the marathon.

Our comment   Complete muscle recovery after marathon racing takes longer than most believe. At some stage in every athlete's career, recovery is incomplete, and their marathon performance suffers as a result. In most great marathon runners, this process is evident after their third to sixth marathon, although there are exceptions such as Katrin Dorre, who ran her fastest marathon at her 30th attempt (see page 61).

The only proven way to speed muscle recovery after marathon racing is to rest. The role of massage, stretching and ice baths in muscle recovery has not been studied, but the widespread acceptance of these techniques by elite athletes, like the great Norwegian marathoner Grete Waitz, suggest that they have value.

---

the first sign of re-injury, one goes immediately for more 'crucifixions'. A little treatment early on in these injuries saves a great deal of agony later.

In order to prevent chronic muscle injuries it is important that the eccentric strength of the muscles at risk of injury is increased and maintained with the appropriate eccentric strengthening programme.

Muscle cramps

Diagnosis

Muscle cramps are defined as spasmodic, painful, involuntary contractions of muscles. Although muscle cramping is an important feature of some very serious muscle disorders, the cramps experienced by runners are, despite the inconvenience and discomfort they cause, usually of little medical consequence. It is clear that the propensity for cramping differs from one individual to another. Some are almost never affected, others will always develop muscle cramps if they run far enough.

Cause
Exertional cramps tend to occur in people who run further or faster than they are accustomed. Thus the athlete whose longest regular training run is 30 km, is likely to develop muscle cramps during the last few kilometres of a 42,2 km standard marathon. University of Cape Town Sports Medicine specialist, Dr Martin Schwellnus, has produced some very convincing evidence that muscle cramps result from alterations in the sensitivity of the reflexes that originate from the muscle and tendon tension receptors. (See physiology of stretching page 44.) It is postulated that during prolonged exercise the inverse stretch reflex, the one that inhibits excessive muscle contraction, becomes inactive. The result is that without this protective reflex, the muscle can go into spasm.

Treatment
The above suggests that the only factor that appears to reduce the risk of cramping is simply more training, especially long-distance runs in those who run marathon and longer races. Adequate pre-race stretching, attention to adequate fluid and carbohydrate replacement before and during exercise, and not running too fast too early in the race, may also be of value. Furthermore the Schwellnus theory predicts that cramps should be prevented if the activity of the inverse stretch reflex is maintained during prolonged exercise. This is done by regularly stretching the tendons of the affected muscles. This stretching reactivates the dormant inverse stretch reflex.

Prevention
The most effective form of prevention for cramps is to undertake a regular stretching programme that focuses especially on the muscles that are prone to cramp during exercise. This programme should incorporate static stretching of the affected muscles for at least ten minutes a day for at least a month. Thereafter it is probable that the benefits can be maintained by a less intensive programme, perhaps ten to fifteen minutes every second day.

Mark Plaatjes *(United States of America)*

Born ninth out of ten children in Coronationville, Johannesburg in 1961, Plaatjes has excelled at distance running in South Africa and the USA. Began competitive running late in secondary school, but immediately focused on long distance events. His first race was over 50 km! Still aged seventeen, he won the SA Marathon title in 2:17:10 at 1800 metres altitude. Completed two year sports scholarship at Georgia University, USA, in early 1980s before returning to South Africa to study physiotherapy. Won SA Marathon Championship in 1985 in 2:08:58.

Also won SA Cross-Country title in that year. Left South Africa in January 1988 for America, where he has become a citizen. Placed third at 1988 Los Angeles Marathon in 2:10:41 and won the Columbus Marathon in 2:12:18 later in that year. Won 1990 Los Angeles Marathon title. Climax of career was the marathon gold medal for the USA at the World Championships at Stuttgart in 1993.

Interview

The most important element of a successful running career is staying injury-free. This allows for consistent progression in training load and gradual improvement in performance. The key to my staying injury-free is listening to my body, regular and consistent stretching and a flexible training programme.

I have been very fortunate in that I have only had niggling injuries that have not kept me out of running for long. These were all muscle or tendon injuries which resulted from similar errors and responded to similar treatment. The injuries were hamstring strain, rectus femoris tendonitis and achilles tendonitis and were all caused through inadequate stretching and not listening to warning signals my body was giving me.

The treatment in all cases consisted of deep friction massage, ultrasound, inferential therapy, icing and regular stretching. In all cases the injury cleared up after three physiotherapy sessions.

Our comment

Mark Plaatjes' victory in the marathon in the 1993 World Championships at Stuttgart was remarkable because it came seven years after he had run his fastest marathon of 2:08:58 in 1985.

Plaatjes' careful approach to his training, and his ability to remain injury-free, have been crucial to his success. Clearly, his medical training as a physiotherapist has provided him with important information. But all the knowledge in the world is useless if the athlete lacks the discipline and courage to resist the urge to train when the body requires caution. In the final analysis, Plaatje's considerable success is built on a mind that is as disciplined and directed as his body is strong and skilful.

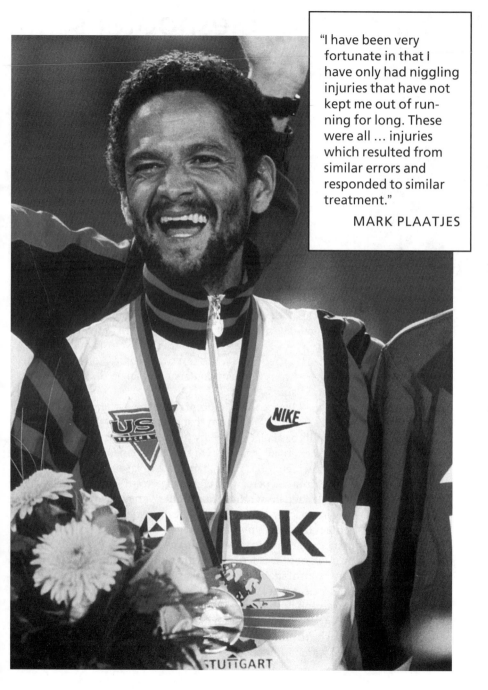

"I have been very fortunate in that I have only had niggling injuries that have not kept me out of running for long. These were all ... injuries which resulted from similar errors and responded to similar treatment."

MARK PLAATJES

7 A troubleshooter's guide

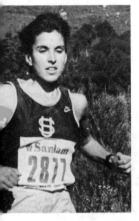

A discussion of site-specific injuries

Injury sites and injury frequency

This should be read in conjunction with the chart on page 162.

It is interesting to know which injuries are the most common. Ligament to bone and tendon to bone attachments appear to be the most vulnerable to injury in runners. Ligaments are non-elastic linkages between bones in a joint, while tendons are non-elastic linkages between muscle and bone. Bones themselves are the next most frequently injured sites, followed by muscles, tendons, bursae (fluid-filled sacs that lie between tendons and bones and allow free movement of the tendons over the bones), bloodvessels (arteries and veins) and nerves. The knee is by far the commonest site of injury, followed by the lower leg with its frequent fibular and tibial bone strain problems ('shinsplints').

A major change that has occurred in the pattern of running injuries since 1970 has been that the incidence of achilles tendonitis has fallen markedly (from about twenty percent to five percent of all injuries). On the other hand, two injuries whose incidence has risen sharply are tibial and fibular bone strain (from ten percent to eighteen percent) and especially peripatellar pain syndrome or runner's knee (from twenty-three percent to forty-four percent). The decrease in the occurrence of achilles tendonitis may be a result of the increased heel height in modern running shoes and increased time spent stretching by modern runners. Also, and probably most importantly, it may be attributable to the softer shoes that are now available. It is now clear that the achilles tendon plays a major role in shock absorption in the lower limb. The reason why the incidence of the other injuries has risen may be due to the same reason, namely, the introduction of softer running shoes which control pronation rather poorly.

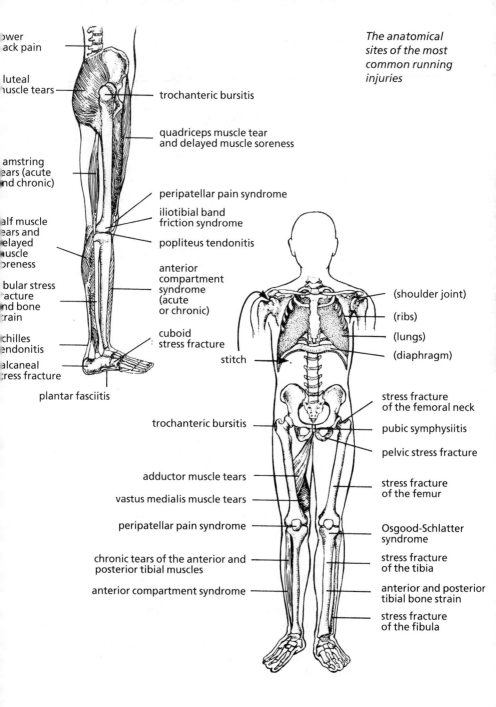

The anatomical sites of the most common running injuries

lower back pain

gluteal muscle tears

trochanteric bursitis

quadriceps muscle tear and delayed muscle soreness

hamstring tears (acute and chronic)

peripatellar pain syndrome

iliotibial band friction syndrome

popliteus tendonitis

calf muscle tears and delayed muscle soreness

anterior compartment syndrome (acute or chronic)

fibular stress fracture and bone strain

cuboid stress fracture

Achilles tendonitis

calcaneal stress fracture

plantar fasciitis

stitch

(shoulder joint)

(ribs)

(lungs)

(diaphragm)

stress fracture of the femoral neck

trochanteric bursitis

pubic symphysiitis

pelvic stress fracture

adductor muscle tears

vastus medialis muscle tears

stress fracture of the femur

peripatellar pain syndrome

Osgood-Schlatter syndrome

chronic tears of the anterior and posterior tibial muscles

stress fracture of the tibia

anterior compartment syndrome

anterior and posterior tibial bone strain

stress fracture of the fibula

A troubleshooter's guide **89**

Upper torso

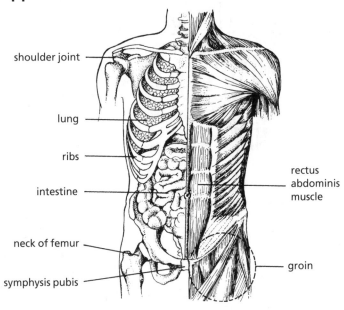

shoulder joint

lung

ribs

intestine

neck of femur

symphysis pubis

rectus
abdominis
muscle

groin

The stitch

Although not an injury to the musculo-skeletal system, the
stitch can prove a debilitating handicap. Many races have been
lost and won through an athlete's ability to endure or get rid of
what can be an excruciatingly painful injury. One of South
Africa's leading distance athletes, Ewald Bonzet, was unable to
race beyond 3 km in the early part of his career because of the
onset of a severe stitch after this distance. He restricted himself
to mile races until he learnt, through breathing techniques, to
overcome this disability.

Diagnosis

The stitch is a condition that occurs only during exercise. It
causes severe pain, usually on the right side of the abdomen
immediately below the rib margin. Pain is also often felt in the
right shoulder joint. The pain is exacerbated by downhill
running and by fast, sustained running. It disappears immediately one lies down. Lying down therefore confirms the
diagnosis.

Cause

Although there is little certainty as to the cause of the stitch, the most likely explanation follows from the Schwellnus theory of muscle cramping (see page 85).

The Schwellnus theory predicts that the stitch, which is a cramp of the diaphragm muscle, occurs because of a loss of the inverse stretch reflex in the diaphragm. This happens, especially during very fast running, because the runner tends to 'pant' or breathe very rapidly without exhaling fully. The result is that the diaphragm is never fully stretched as it would be during a full exhalation, and consequently the inverse stretch reflex is not activated. The diaphragm therefore goes into spasm because the inverse stretch reflex is not functioning.

It used to be believed that the stitch developed from the diaphragm becoming 'trapped' between an over-expanded chest (resulting from shallow breathing) and a jolting intestine below. This, it was said, caused the diaphragm to go into spasm.

Treatment

If the stitch develops during a race there are two measures that frequently help.

One is to alter the breathing pattern so that one breathes out when landing on the foot opposite the side where the pain is; the other is to exhale forcefully and fully (grunt) with each breath. This re-stretches the diaphragm and reactivates the inverse stretch reflex.

Prevention, however, is always preferable to cure. There is empirical, if not scientific, evidence to suggest that 'belly-breathing' (breathing mainly with the diaphragm) can prevent the onset of the stitch.

To learn to belly-breathe, lie on your back with a large book on your stomach. The book should rise when you breathe in and fall as the air is expelled from your lungs. It takes about two months to learn to belly-breathe while running at speed.

Increasing abdominal muscle strength can also help prevent the onset of the stitch. The correct way to do this is to do bent-knee sit-ups with the feet unsupported.

The way to prevent the stitch during racing is to ensure that you exhale fully. One or two very large and complete exhalations, in which the diaphragm is stretched to its greatest extent, can break the stitch almost instantaneously.

Back

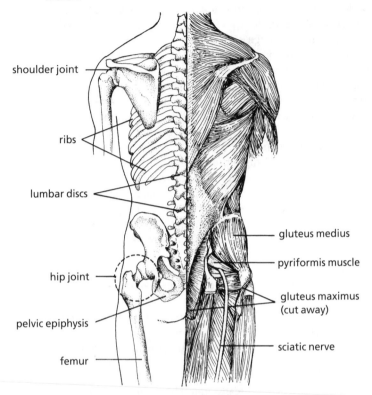

shoulder joint

ribs

lumbar discs

gluteus medius

pyriformis muscle

hip joint

gluteus maximus
(cut away)

pelvic epiphysis

sciatic nerve

femur

Low back pain including sciatica

Something like seventy percent of all adults complain of
moderate or severe low back pain and the management of this
condition in anyone, runners included, is a very specialized area
of medicine. Runners with this complaint are advised to consult
only specialists who have expert knowledge in this field.

Low back pain in runners can arise from three primary
sources:

☐ Through degeneration of the discs between the vertebrae in
the lower back.
☐ From a stress fracture of the segment (the pars interarticu-
laris) of the vertebrae spanning the spinal cord. This is an
uncommon injury in runners but more common in sports in
which there is twisting of the spine, for example, fast
bowling in cricket.

☐ Through injury to other tissues, for example, ligaments, muscles and the small joints of the back. Of these, the first two are the more serious.

If the intervertebral disc protrudes into the spinal canal it may cause pressure on the nerves in the canal, especially the sciatic nerve. When this happens the runner feels pain not only in the back but also along the distribution of the sciatic nerve in the lower leg. This condition is known as sciatica and indicates that the back injury is more serious and requires more careful management.

Occasionally low back pain is due to more sinister diseases, like cancer that has spread from its initial site. This must always be considered, especially in older people.

Diagnosis

Pain which shoots from the back and passes through the buttocks, down the back of the thigh and possibly to the foot is indicative of sciatica (pressure on or damage to the sciatic nerve). Pain when lifting an unbent leg while lying down is also suggestive of this ailment. General low back pain which does not respond to conventional treatment (see below) could indicate the more serious disc degeneration. Just occasionally the 'low back pain' is nothing more than pain referred from chronic buttock muscle tears.

An important characteristic is that sciatica occurs only in people who also have low back pain or discomfort at other times of the day, when they are not exercising. 'Low back pain' or 'sciatica' that occurs only during exercise is due to something other than damage to vertebral discs.

Cause

There is some evidence that a disproportionate number of joggers and cross-country skiers complain of moderate low back pain. This is probably due in part to:

☐ the loading on the back during running;
☐ strength imbalances between the abdominal and back muscles;
☐ inflexibility of the hamstring muscles.

Pain may also be aggravated if there is an associated short-leg syndrome or ankle pronation during running.

It would seem that the worst physical activities for the back

Colleen de Reuck (see page 33)

Interview   *I began running again about four weeks after giving birth to Tamsyn. I think a combination of sleep deprivation and breast feeding might have weakened my ligaments and led to my pelvis being pulled slightly out of alignment. This is turn pulled on my muscles in my back, causing pain. The fact that I was unable to take anti-inflammatory tablets as I was breast-feeding exacerbated the problem.*

Fortunately I was not pressurized to get back to competition and I was able to do so in my own time, taking more time (an extra two months) than was necessary. The back pain vanished about five months after birth, which coincided with Tamsyn being weaned.

Our comment   Low back pain is a common complaint in the latter stages of pregnancy and also shortly after giving birth, for all the reasons that Colleen de Reuck describes. Rest and a gradual return to training will allow the normal physiological changes of pregnancy to reverse, and the associated low back discomfort to disappear.

---

are those encountered in work activities that involve weight lifting, in particular those which combine weight lifting with twisting of the spine. Jogging and other leisure activities may increase the symptoms of moderate, but not severe, low back pain. Paradoxically, lack of fitness is strongly associated with an increased incidence of low back pain.

Sciatica can be aggravated by hill running. Overstriding associated with downhill running increases impact shock, which is transferred to the damaged disc. The tightening of the gluteal muscles (see diagram page 92) associated with uphill running can have the same effect.

Treatment

Treatment of low back pain in a runner is a very specialized area requiring careful evaluation of the injury and, where appropriate, the prescription of suitable low back exercises. Stretching the gluteal muscles can also be helpful. This should

be done in conjunction with abdominal strengthening exercises aimed at redressing muscle strength and flexibility imbalances.

Good posture will guard against back pain and runners who already suffer low back pain should try to improve their posture. In this regard yoga exercises and, in particular, lessons in the Alexander technique can be helpful. All this advice can be acquired from a knowledgeable physiotherapist, Alexander technique instructor, or yoga instructor, who should be consulted as early as possible.

If you have severe lumbar disc degeneration, should you undergo surgery? Here again the general advice is that surgery should always be delayed for as long as possible. However, if it turns out that surgery is necessary, the good news is that in runners at least, the results are frequently successful.

Buttocks

Chronic tears of the buttock muscles

Diagnosis
Pain caused by chronic tears of the pyriformis or gluteal muscles (see diagram page 92) is quite easily diagnosed because runners will complain of discomfort in the buttock and will usually be able to localize the site of discomfort to the affected muscle. Pain may be associated with restricted forward movement of the hip on the affected side. These injuries could, however, be confused with sciatica. The diagnosis is confirmed by finding the tender knot, using the technique described on page 80.

Cause
As with other chronic tears the mechanism of injury is unknown, but it is probably related to the high degree of loading (external force) applied to a small section of the muscle as a result of high quantity and/or quality training. This is more fully explained on page 81.

Treatment
The only effective treatment consists of vigorous cross-frictions (page 82) and appropriate stretching exercises (page 50 and 54).

Olga Appell *(United States of America)*

Born in Mexico. Began running at twenty-four in 1987 to lose weight after birth of daughter, Monique. Moved to Germany for three years with husband and coach, Brian, before returning to Albuquerque in the USA. Placed second (1:08:34) in 1992 Tokyo Half-Marathon to Elana Meyer. Won Long Beach and Sapporo Marathons in 1992 and Los Angeles (2:28:12, PB) and Hokaido Marathons in 1994. Placed second in New York Marathon in 2:32:45 in 1994. Reached the 10 000 m finals at the World Track Championships in 1993 and in 1994 won the American 10 000 m title in 32:03. Set USA 12 km record of 38:45 in 1994 and was rated No. 3 in the world in that year behind Elana Meyer in *Running Times'* rating of distance running. Second American home at the 1995 World Cross-Country Championships in 14th position.

Interview

After running a personal best at the Tokyo Half-Marathon in 1992, I immediately caught a flight home. It was a long flight and I believe that being cramped up after the race was partly responsible for my injury, which started playing up on my return. I had a pain in my low back and buttocks and I could not run for longer than fifteen minutes before being forced to stop.

Original chiropractic and massage treatment failed to work, but then a physiotherapist friend applied deep cross-frictions to the painful site. It was excruciating, but after two sessions I could run again and after three I was free of pain.

I tried racing shortly after Gaspirilla (15 km), but the injury recurred and forced me to drop out. I had another three cross-friction sessions (about five to six weeks after the injury first occurred) and since then (for three and a half years) I have had no pain.

I try to run off tarmac wherever possible, and stretch after my training runs. It does not always happen, though, and I know I should stretch more often.

Our comment

Appell's experience with deep cross-friction therapy is typical: despite the pain, it is the only effective treatment for chronic muscle tears. Therapy should always be continued until running is again pain-free. These injuries tend to recur, and physiotherapy should be used to treat each recurrence as soon as the pain develops again. Delaying treatment slows recovery.

Hip, pelvis and groin

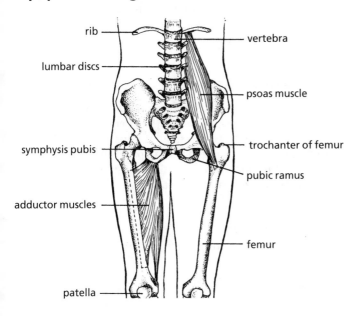

Labels (clockwise from top left): rib, lumbar discs, symphysis pubis, adductor muscles, patella, femur, pubic ramus, trochanter of femur, psoas muscle, vertebra

Chronic muscle tears of the adductor muscles

Diagnosis
Chronic muscle tears of the adductor muscles in the groin (see diagram above) are diagnosed in the same way as all other chronic muscle tears (see page 80). Pain begins gradually, allowing the athlete to run through it, but worsens progressively. Although the immediate pain subsides with rest, this form of treatment is ineffective in healing the injury, which recurs immediately the athlete begins to run. On palpation of the painful area, a tender knot is felt.

Cause
The injury is due to an abnormally high loading of the specific muscle site as a result of high quality (speed) or high quantity (distance) training.

Treatment
Vigorous cross-frictions are the only effective treatment.

Chronic muscle tears of the psoas muscle

This muscle is located high up on the front of the thigh (see diagram page 97) and the diagnosis and cause of this injury are the same as for other chronic muscle tears (see page 80).

Diagnosis

The following symptoms indicate the injury:

- [ ] As with any chronic muscle tear, the onset of pain is gradual. The pain is usually nagging rather than debilitating.
- [ ] The pain eases rapidly with rest but returns with exercise.
- [ ] The contraction of the muscle causes pain. This can be done by lying face-up and flexing the hip against resistance.
- [ ] The injury is tender to the touch and a knot can be felt at the site of pain.

Cause and treatment

These are the same as for the hamstring injury on page 102.

Stress fracture of the pelvis

Diagnosis

A stress fracture of the pelvis (see diagram page 97) may initially be confused with a chronic adductor muscle tear. At first there is ill-defined discomfort in the groin but, in contrast to a muscle tear, if the athlete continues to run the discomfort soon becomes so severe that running is impossible. When this occurs, the diagnosis of a stress fracture is no longer in doubt.

An important diagnostic feature is the 'standing test'. Athletes with a pelvic stress fracture experience pain or discomfort in the groin when asked to put all their weight on the injured leg. It is believed that this symptom is not present in any other injury. Many first notice this symptom when they try to put on under-clothes or trousers. They cannot do this standing only on the leg on the affected side, so they begin to sit down when dressing.

Cause

The mechanism of injury in this fracture is unknown but it almost certainly involves abnormal shearing stresses across the pelvis, of the same kind that cause osteitis pubis (see page 97 and page 100). It is of interest that the injury is far more common among women than among men and seems to affect women who train hardest, who are the most competitive and who may have amenorrhoea (absence of normal menstruation).

Treatment
As with all stress fractures, the only treatment is rest. This particular fracture usually takes between eight to twelve weeks to heal properly but there have been cases where the injury has taken up to twenty-three weeks to heal completely. Everyday walking loads the injured site and delays healing. Thus even walking should be restricted at first, until it can be done without causing discomfort.

Stress fracture of the neck of the femur

Diagnosis
The diagnosis of this uncommon injury is often overlooked or delayed. However, this a potentially serious injury.

Femoral neck stress fractures cause pain in the front of the hip and, as for almost all fractures, the pain is always so severe that running is impossible. This is a serious fracture because the fracture line crosses the bloodvessels that keep the head of the femur, the part that fits into the hip joint, alive. If the bloodvessels are severely damaged, the head of the femur may die because its blood supply has been interrupted. Death of the head of the femur will ultimately lead to osteoarthritis of the hip and severe disability in later life.

Alternatively, the fracture may move out of its normal anatomical alignment (displace) and lead to a fracture that either does not heal (non-union) or heals in the incorrect alignment (malunion).

For this reason, pain in the front of the hip that prevents running must be taken very seriously and must be evaluated immediately by an orthopaedic surgeon. The fracture frequently fails to show on X-ray so that a bone scan may be required. Even then, the fracture may not show. Thus the diagnosis must often be made solely on clinical grounds. Many runners correctly diagnose their own injury.

Treatment
There is little consensus as to how this injury should be treated, although it has been suggested it should be treated on the basis of the radiological changes. This would involve a range of treatment, depending on evidence from the X-rays, varying from

allowing the patient to walk with crutches (to avoid bearing weight), through bed rest to emergency pinning of the fracture in hospital. These decisions can be made only by an orthopaedic surgeon. If you think you have this fracture, consult an ortho-paedic surgeon urgently. But don't let the surgeon dismiss your symptoms unless he or she has read this section of the book!

Pubic symphysiitis

Pubic symphysiitis or osteitis pubis is an ill-defined injury in which the athlete complains of pain over the symphysis pubis (see diagram page 97), often at the point of attachment of the large muscles that form the anterior (front) abdominal wall.

Diagnosis

The following are the most important diagnostic features:

☐ Pain in the pubis, which can be severe. Turning over while lying down sometimes reproduces the pain in the lower stomach or groin.

☐ Typically the pain comes on after one has run a set distance, and persists until one stops running. Usually the pain has a nagging, annoying quality, but it seldom becomes severe enough to prevent running completely.

☐ Sit-ups and coughing especially reproduce the pain.

☐ On palpation of the symphysis pubis, marked tenderness is reproduced.

☐ On X-ray there are specific radiological features that suggest the diagnosis.

Cause

The cause of the injury is unknown but it probably involves the same shearing forces across the joint (due to lower limb abnor-mality) that cause pelvic stress fractures and adductor muscle tears. It appears to be an injury of more experienced runners — that is, those who have exposed their skeletons to high loading over many years.

Treatment

There is no known effective way to treat this injury. The approach should be to correct any overt biomechanical lower limb abnormalities, but in some cases, surgery may have to be the ultimate resort. Cortisone injections into the tender area have also been used but their effectiveness has not been proven.

Some physiotherapists practise a technique, described in *Lore of Running*, for this injury which involves the mobilization of the symphysis pubis. Whether or not this technique will prove to be any more effective than others for the treatment of this injury is unknown. However, given that this is an injury which stubbornly resists most forms of treatment, it is probably worth a try. Prolonged rest of six to twelve months may be the only effective treatment for this condition.

Trochanteric bursitis

Bursae are fluid-filled sacs that prevent tendons rubbing directly on bone. The trochanteric bursa lies between the trochanter of the femur and the iliotibial band (page 106). Trochanteric bursitis is the inflammation of this bursa. Although relatively uncommon, there are two other sites at which bursitis can develop. These are on the inside of the knee (pes anerinus busitis) and the retrocalcaneal bursa between the heel (calcaneal) bone and the achilles tendon.

Diagnosis

When inflamed, the bursa causes pain to be felt over the bony trochanter at the side of the leg. This condition is known as trochanteric bursitis.

The pain is reproduced by having the runner lie on his or her side, injured side up. Abducting (moving sideways away from the midline) and flexing the hip while applying pressure to the trochanter reproduces the pain.

Cause

The causes of trochanteric bursistis are probably the same as the causes of the iliotibial band friction syndrome (see page 113). The major factors are summarized below:

☐ Heavy training distances, a sudden increase in training and/or too much racing
☐ Excessive downhill running or running on hard surfaces
☐ Running predominantly on one side of a cambered road
☐ Hard running shoes with low shock-absorbing potential
☐ Rigid 'clunk' feet (see page 19)

Treatment

The treatment is essentially the same as for the iliotibial band friction syndrome. This consists of prescription of soft running

Eamonn Martin (see page 31)

Interview *In 1985 and 1986 I battled with an extremely painful achilles, which made running highly uncomfortable and thwarted any serious competitive running in those years. In the end I decided on surgery to remove an inflamed bursa behind the achilles tendon, which proved successful. It was important, though, to look at the biomechanical reasons for having suffered the injury, and my pronation deficiencies were corrected with orthotics.*

Our comment Martin confirms the value of using orthotics to prevent the recurrence of chronic injuries, including achilles tendonitis and plantar fasciitis. It appears that he suffered retrocalcaneal bursitis and that surgery effectively cured that injury.

shoes from which the lateral heel-flare has been removed; lateral stretching exercises (see exercise 14 on page 54); and, most importantly, shoe modifications to compensate for any leg-length inequalities. A single cortisone injection into the bursa, given by an experienced orthopaedic surgeon, is often particularly effective.

Trochanteric bursitis is usually associated with a chronic muscle tear of the tensor fascia lata muscle (see diagram page 106). This inserts into the iliotibial band immediately above the trochanter of the femur. In cases of trochanteric bursitis, this muscle should always be examined. If a chronic muscle tear is found, it must be treated with vigorous cross-frictions by a physiotherapist.

Upper Leg
Chronic hamstring tear
Much of the discussion on chronic muscle tears from page 80 onwards is applicable since muscle tears have similarities regardless of site.

Diagnosis
The following are the diagnostic features for the chronic hamstring tear:

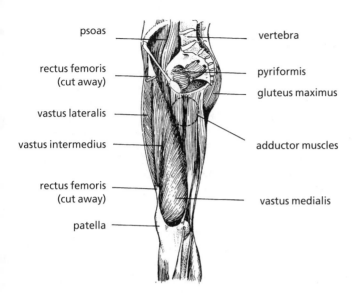

psoas

vertebra

rectus femoris
(cut away)

pyriformis

gluteus maximus

vastus lateralis

vastus intermedius

adductor muscles

rectus femoris
(cut away)

vastus medialis

patella

☐ As with any chronic muscle tear, the onset of pain is gradual. The description of the pain is usually nagging rather than debilitating.

☐ The pain passes off rapidly with rest but recurs during exercise. Walking and standing do not reproduce the symptoms. When the pain is present, the athlete may find it difficult to extend the knee on the affected side easily or rapidly.

☐ Unlike true sciatica or general low back pain, no symptoms are felt when one is not running.

☐ Bending forwards with straightened legs can reproduce the pain. (This has the effect of stretching the hamstrings.)

☐ A tender knot, which may be deep-seated, can be felt in the painful area of the hamstring muscle.

☐ The pain may appear to move to two or three sites during the healing process.

Cause

The hamstring tear, like any other chronic muscle tear, is probably the result of the specific small site of the muscle being subjected to abnormally high loading (application of forces) as a result of an increase in quality or quantity of training.

Remember that the muscle tears when contracting eccentrically.

Sonja Laxton *(South Africa)*

In a class of her own as a veteran distance athlete in SA, she was forty-six when she competed in the 1994 World Half-Marathon Championships in Oslo as a senior — the oldest in the field. She clocked 1:16:46. Has run competitively since she was fifteen, when she was limited to 220 yards as the longest distance women were allowed to run. Moved to 800 m at seventeen, then won senior 1500 m title aged twenty-two. Frequently chosen to represent SA in track, cross-country and road. Won SA's first marathon title for women in 1981 at thirty-two and won it again in 1993 at forty-four. Set national marathon record of 2:35:44 in 1986. PBs for 10 km, 15 km and half-marathon of 34:02, 51:45 and 1:13:45.

Interview

I think the problem arose when I was doing aerobics. We had to do those stretches on the ballet bars — raising your leg at ninety degrees. I think my hamstring was just too tight and it tore.

I was off competition for about six months from August 1985 and missed the 1986 marathon championships as a result.

I went to fourteen different specialists. Seven thought the problem was my sciatic nerve, while the other half identified it as a hamstring injury, which it proved to be.

At first it was difficult to pinpoint the exact spot as the pain seemed to move every time! Finally they did locate it and from November 1985 I began to receive cross-friction treatment from a physiotherapist. Although this was extremely painful I was able to return to training within six weeks and so far I have not had a recurrence of the injury.

Our comment

Sonja's story of a chronic hamstring tear is typical: it is an injury that is often missed by medical doctors, including orthopaedic surgeons, because it is poorly described in the medical textbooks and is not taught in those medical schools that do not have a strong interest in sports medicine.

Cross-frictioning (deep transverse friction massage) is the only effective treatment for this condition. If the cross-frictions are not as painful as Sonja describes them, then either the diagnosis is incorrect or the wrong muscle is being treated.

Hamstring injuries continue to be an important cause of disability, especially in elite runners like Sonja Laxton and David Tsebe who include a high proportion of speedwork in their training. These injuries become chronic as a result of scarring within muscles that are repeatedly damaged. Each instance of injury increases the probability that the injury will become more prone to re-injury, and more resistant to cure.

Thus, each episode of injury should be treated properly. In addition heavy training, especially speedwork, should recommence only when the injury is fully healed and rehabilitated.

Although eccentric muscle strengthening is currently under-utilized by most athletes with muscle injuries, it is likely that this will prove to be an essential form of treatment (see page 84).

Treatment

The only effective treatment is physiotherapy in the form of a series of cross-friction treatments. Ultrasound application following the cross-frictions may aid the healing process. Long-term prevention requires that the eccentric strength of the hamstring muscles be increased. This requires the supervision of a physiotherapist or exercise rehabilitation specialist.

Chronic muscle tears of the quadriceps muscles

These are muscles of the front of the thigh (see diagram page 106) and the diagnosis, cause and treatment of tears to these muscles is essentially the same as for chronic tears to any muscle.

Diagnosis

The following symptoms indicate the injury:

☐ As with any chronic muscle tear, the onset of pain is gradual. The description of the pain is usually nagging rather than debilitating. When pain is present the athlete may experience difficulty in extending the knee.
☐ The pain passes rapidly with rest but recurs during exercise.
☐ The contraction of these muscles causes pain. This can be achieved by lying on one's back and flexing the knee.
☐ The injury is tender to the touch and a knot may be felt at the site of pain.

Cause and treatment

The cause of the injury and its treatment are the same as for the chronic tear of the hamstring discussed above.

Acute muscle tear of the hamstring muscle

The acute (sudden) muscle tear is the classic muscle injury of sprinting, which involves explosive muscle contractions not normally associated with distance running.

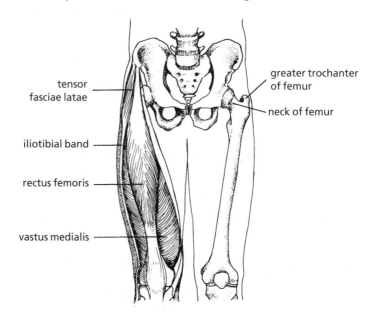

tensor fasciae latae

greater trochanter of femur

neck of femur

iliotibial band

rectus femoris

vastus medialis

Diagnosis

The athlete is suddenly overcome by agonizingly severe pain in the affected muscle; there is immediate loss of function. The muscle is in spasm, is extremely tender and over the next few hours swells. The skin overlying the injury may show bruising.

Cause

Acute muscle tears are believed to result from a combination of the following factors: inadequate eccentric strength of the affected hamstring; muscle strength imbalance between opposing muscle groups; inflexibility of the affected muscles; and inadequate warm-up.

One theory is that the sprinter's hamstring tear is caused by an activity (very fast running) which overdevelops the front thigh muscles (quadriceps) at the expense of the hamstrings, which become correspondingly weaker. When this strength imbalance reaches a critical value, the quadriceps literally overpowers the hamstring, causing a severe muscle tear.

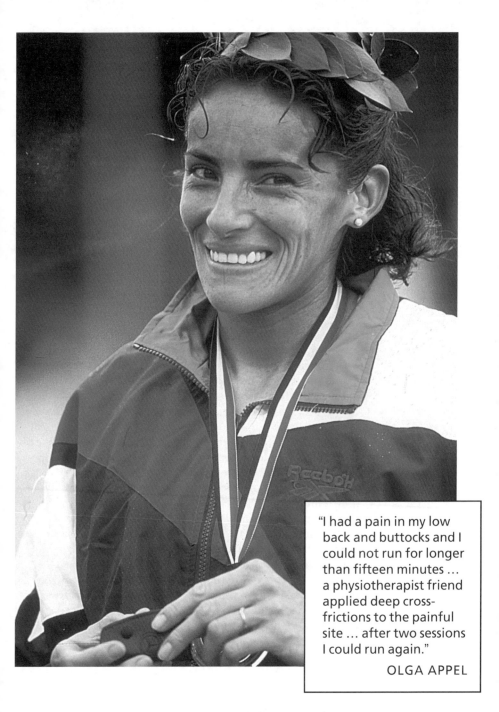

"I had a pain in my low back and buttocks and I could not run for longer than fifteen minutes ... a physiotherapist friend applied deep cross-frictions to the painful site ... after two sessions I could run again."

OLGA APPEL

A troubleshooter's guide   107

Alternatively, sprint training itself may not develop the eccentric strength of the hamstring muscles sufficiently. They then become too weak to cope with the increased loading caused by very fast running.

Treatment

The immediate treatment of the acute muscle tear is to apply ice to the tender area without delay, to rest and elevate the injured limb and to apply a firm compression bandage over the site of the tear as soon as the initial ice application is completed.

Athletes below eighteen years of age should be seen by an orthopaedic surgeon to check that they have not pulled off the pelvic epiphysis. This is the end of the bone which, in children, is separated from its shaft by a cartilaginous growth plate; the hamstring muscles are attached to it.

Next, and most important, comes specific treatment and early rehabilitation.

A serious acute muscle tear is often considered to be such a severe injury that rest for six to eight weeks is desirable. However, benefit can be derived from an intensive regime involving vigorous treatment of the injured muscle together with muscle stretching and strengthening for as many as six half-hour sessions a day, beginning forty-eight hours after injury. It has been shown that this can return most athletes with serious acute muscle injuries to competitive sport within ten to fourteen days.

The critical issue in acute muscle injuries, particularly those of the hamstring, is to prevent their recurrence. This can be done only if the muscle balance is corrected by strengthening the hamstrings. This can be achieved by running longer distances — unlike sprinting, distance running develops primarily the hamstrings, not the quadriceps. Alternatively, one can try specific muscle-strengthening exercises performed on an isokinetic machine under expert supervision. Eccentric strengthening must also be emphasized.

Hamstring stretching (see page 48 and after) should also be performed religiously, also under supervision, and no fast running must be undertaken, unless there has been an adequate warm-up and the hamstring to quadriceps strength ratio is correct. Fast running must always be avoided in cold conditions.

Stress fracture of the shaft of the femur

This injury accounts for two per cent of all stress fractures. The diagnosis, cause and treatment are essentially as discussed in the section on stress fractures in general on page 68.

Delayed muscle soreness and cramping of the quadriceps and hamstrings

The diagnosis, cause and treatment of these injuries has been adequately dealt with under the general discussion of muscle injuries beginning on page 77.

Knee

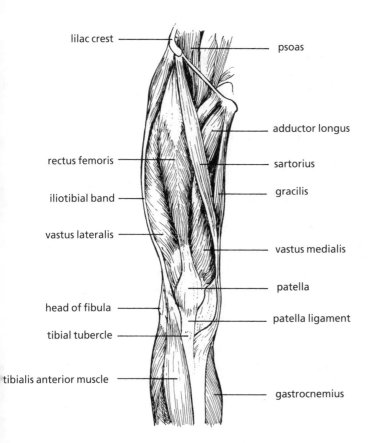

lilac crest

psoas

adductor longus

rectus femoris

sartorius

gracilis

iliotibial band

vastus lateralis

vastus medialis

patella

head of fibula

patella ligament

tibial tubercle

tibialis anterior muscle

gastrocnemius

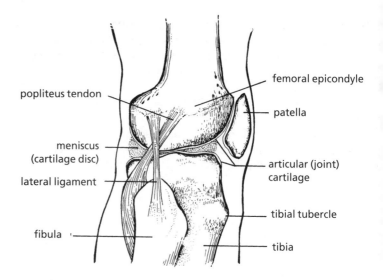

*View from
lateral side*

popliteus tendon

femoral epicondyle

patella

meniscus
(cartilage disc)

lateral ligament

articular (joint)
cartilage

tibial tubercle

fibula

tibia

Peripatellar pain syndrome ('runner's knee')

The term 'runner's knee' was first coined by Dr George Sheehan
in the early 1970s to describe a running injury that produces a
set of very specific and characteristic symptoms.

In the original description of runner's knee, it was thought
that the damaged tissues in this injury lay behind the kneecap
in the cartilaginous lining of the knee joint. Thus runner's knee
was considered to be chondromalacia patella — a condition well
recognized by orthopaedic surgeons and in which there is
degeneration of the joint cartilage on the undersurface of the
kneecap.

If this were indeed the case it would mean that running had
caused degeneration of the joint cartilage which, in time, would
almost certainly lead to arthritis. We now know that runner's
knee is not chondromalacia patella and that it has nothing to
do with the cartilage lining the undersurface of the kneecap.
Rather, the condition should be called 'peripatellar pain
syndrome' to indicate that the injury involves the structures
around the kneecap, in particular the ligamentous attachments
at the lower end of the patella. The injury is also known as
medial retinaculitis or patellofemoral pain syndrome.

Studies have shown this injury to be the most common of all
those associated with distance running.

Diagnosis

The following are pointers to the diagnosis of the injury:

- ☐ The pain is localized around the kneecap, usually at the lower end.
- ☐ The pain first occurs during running and does not result from external trauma.
- ☐ The pain usually comes on after running a predictable distance.
- ☐ The pain becomes gradually worse, but is exacerbated by very long races.
- ☐ Walking up or down steps causes discomfort, as does squatting on the haunches.
- ☐ Sitting with the knee bent for any length of time causes discomfort, which is relieved by straightening (extending) the knee.
- ☐ The conventional medical approach to sporting injuries — cortisone injections into the painful area — never provides a permanent cure. Nor does the surgical procedure in which the cartilage behind the kneecap is 'shaved'.

The diagnosis of peripatellar pain syndrome can be confirmed by a simple test in which the runner lies on his or her back on the examining couch and relaxes the quadriceps (upper thigh) muscle.

The left hand pushes the top end of the patella so that the bottom tip comes away from the knee joint. Firm pressure with the second and third fingers along the lower border of the patella reproduces the pain the athlete feels when running.

Cause

Peripatellar pain syndrome is the injury which, par excellence, is caused by excessive ankle pronation (see structural deficiencies page 18).

The excessive pronation causes a twisting force to develop at the knee (see diagram page 110). This pulls the kneecap out of its correct alignment, causing increased stress on the kneecap-anchoring ligaments, shown on page 109.

With time, this abnormal movement, repeated sufficiently frequently, causes the bone to which the ligaments are attached to develop a stress response, ultimately causing pain.

There are several other factors that may be associated with this injury:

Shoes

Inappropriately soft running shoes which may have collapsed to the inside fail to control pronation adequately and may contribute to the injury (see shoes page 36). Conversely, very hard running shoes may also cause the injury by increasing shock loading at the knee.

Training errors and training surfaces

Other causative factors include training too far, too hard and too soon, always running on the same side of a cambered road, interval training and racing too often. Note that this injury is more likely to occur on the leg nearest to the middle of the road. This is because it is the inside foot that must pronate excessively to compensate for the road camber.

Hereditary factors

The most important hereditary factor causing the ankle to pronate excessively in runners with this injury, is a pair of hypermobile feet. In addition, there may be other abnormalities that cause the kneecap to drift inwards during the stance phase of running (see biomechanics of running page 12), and these include an abnormal inward twist in the femur.

Treatment

The first aid treatment of runner's knee is to apply ice to the sore area for about twenty minutes twice daily. Cortisone injections into the knee joint, although suggested by some writers, must be avoided at all costs as they do not reach the site of the injury which is around the kneecap, not in the knee joint itself. There is also evidence that these injections may predispose to the development of arthritis in later life.

The most important treatment of runner's knee, however, must be aimed at correcting the biomechanical factors causing it, namely excessive ankle pronation. If the biomechanical cause is not corrected, the kneecap will continue to be pulled out of alignment with each running stride and this will successfully defeat all medical efforts that aim simply at treating the painful area on the kneecap. This correction is achieved by running in shoes that limit ankle pronation (see shoes on page 38) and, if this fails to do so and thus cure the injury, by having a custom-built corrective orthotic made.

Unless the corrective orthotic is correctly made, the injury will not improve. Sports podiatry is a relatively new profession and until recently, people sufficiently qualified to make corrective orthotics were difficult to find. Now, however, there are sports podiatrists in most major centres throughout the world. Arch supports that can be bought over the counter at pharmacies and running shoe shops are usually not sufficient for athletes who pronate excessively, although they may help runners with only very mild degrees of abnormal pronation. Injured runners unable to consult a podiatrist would be well-advised first to try using a commercially available arch support such as the Spenco full length arch support.

Other methods of treatment include calf muscle stretching (see exercise no 7 on page 51) and correcting any possible muscle strength and flexibility imbalances between the quadriceps and hamstring muscles.

Runners with this injury who fail to improve within about a month must realize that this is because the shoes and corrective orthotics that they are using have failed to control their ankle pronation sufficiently. Further correction is necessary.

Iliotibial band friction syndrome (ITB)

The iliotibial band is a thickened strip of fascia (tendon) that extends from the hip across the outside of the knee, to insert into the large shin bone, the tibia, immediately below the line of the knee joint (see diagram page 109). When the knee is straight, the fascia lies in front of a bony prominence at the outside of the knee, the femoral epicondyle, but as the knee bends, the fascia begins to move towards that bony point. When the knee has bent through about thirty degrees, the fascia may touch the femoral epicondyle and it is this contact which is believed to cause the pain.

Although not as common as peripatellar pain syndrome, this injury accounts for about a third to a fifth of all knee injuries in distance runners. It is also the injury most resistant to treatment.

Diagnosis

The classic feature of this injury is severe pain, well localized over the outside of the knee, directly over the lateral femoral epicondyle (see diagram page 110). The site is exquisitely tender to pressure. The pain is absent at rest and only comes on during exercise. Even though they may be quite unable to run, athletes are usually able to walk long distances or play other sports, for example, squash, rugby or tennis, without discomfort. However, walking downstairs may be painful.

During running, the pain usually becomes so severe that it limits the runner to a specific running distance which may be as little as 100 m in some and as much as 16 km in others. The pain usually comes on rapidly and then stops further running.

Downhill running, in particular, aggravates the symptoms in all runners. Sometimes, but rarely, symptoms are only present during downhill running; in such cases, runners may be able to continue running on the flat or uphill, avoiding downhills.

Another important feature of this injury is that the pain subsides almost immediately the athlete stops running.

The diagnosis is confirmed by the 'Noble test', in which pressure is applied to the lateral side (outside) of the knee directly over the femoral epicondyle. The knee is slowly straightened from about ninety degrees of flexion. At about thirty degrees of flexion, as the band slips over the femoral epicondyle directly underneath the examiner's finger, the pain that the athlete feels during activity is reproduced. This test may not elicit pain if the runner has not run for the previous three or more days — so be sure to run on the day of the examination.

Cause

At present there is no consensus of how this injury occurs or how it should be treated, but some of the factors that have been isolated include the following:

Training errors

It would seem that heavy training mileages, sudden increases in training and too much racing are important training errors that explain why this injury occurs most commonly in the peak racing season. Alternatively, a heavy training load sustained for many months may cause this injury.

Training surfaces

Excessive downhill running and running on hard surfaces seem to be factors in this injury. Further, the injury occurs on the side of the body corresponding to the side of the road on which the runner most often runs.

Shoes

Hard shoes which are designed to limit ankle pronation and which have poor shock absorption qualities, seem to be a very important causative factor.

Bhekizizwe Willie Mtolo *(South Africa)*

Born May 1964 near Underberg in the southern Drakensberg. One of SA's best-known marathoners abroad, mostly due to his win in the 1992 New York Marathon. Eldest son of family. Could not afford bike so ran 16 km to school barefoot. Substantial physical work on family smallholding. Formed Willie Mtolo Athletics Club to promote running development in region. Best 10 km road time of 28:43 and one second faster on the track. Best 15 km of 43:29. Best half-marathon of 1:01:52. Second in 1986 SA Marathon in his best of 2:08:15. Won SA Marathon titles in 1988 (2:10:18) and 1989. First 1992 New York Marathon (2:09:29), second 1994 Rotterdam (2:10:17), seventh 1995 London (2:11:35).

Interview

I began my running career in Pietermaritzburg, where everyone is focused on one race only — the Comrades Marathon. So naturally I found myself training for that race, which I ran in 1984, finishing in about six hours. [Mtolo placed 23rd in 6:02:40].

I was very inexperienced then and ran many marathons that year, including a few ultra-marathons. Perhaps it was not surprising that I became injured! I developed a pain on the outside of my knee, which was later diagnosed as the ITB.

In spite of treatment I was troubled by the injury on and off for about three years. After my 2:08:15 marathon in Port Elizabeth in 1986 my knee was very painful.

Fortunately since 1988 I have had no further symptoms and I have been virtually injury-free, possibly because I planned my racing schedule more carefully. Although it took me a long while to recover from the Comrades in 1989, it was not due to injury. [Mtolo placed second in 5:39:59].

Our comment

Bhekizizwe Mtolo's biomechanical structures, in which he has a very mild genu varum (bow legs), is such that he is predisposed to develop the iliotibial band syndrome, especially if he runs with hard running shoes on hard running surfaces or includes excessive downhill running in his training.

The fact that Mtolo has been so successful indicates that these biomechanical abnormalities were sufficiently minor in his case to allow the body to compensate for them. But wearing the most appropriate running shoes, and including preventative measures like regular stretching and reducing training when minor aches develop after training, all reduce the risk of subsequent injury. This is true even for runners with near-ideal biomechanical structure.

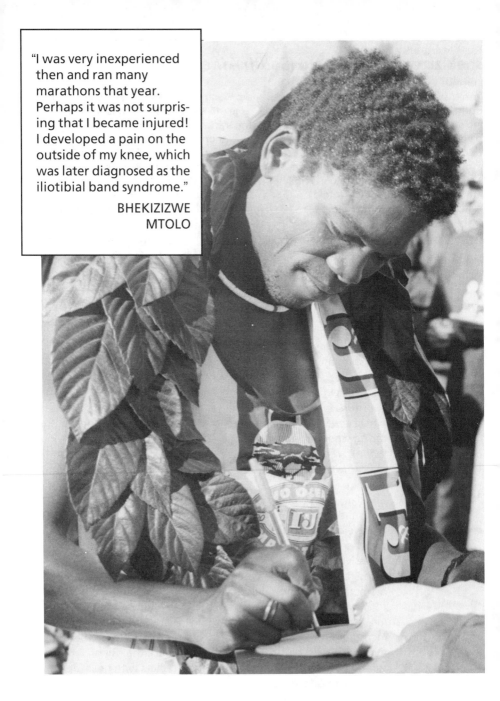

"I was very inexperienced then and ran many marathons that year. Perhaps it was not surprising that I became injured! I developed a pain on the outside of my knee, which was later diagnosed as the iliotibial band syndrome."

BHEKIZIZWE
MTOLO

Hereditary factors

The most important hereditary structural factors associated with this injury are bow-legs and high-arched, rigid feet. Rigid feet are unable to absorb adequately the shock of landing, which is then transferred in some way to the iliotibial band and this ultimately leads to the injury. On the other hand, some runners with extremely flat feet which are also unable to absorb shock adequately may be equally at risk.

Treatment

Treatment must aim to increase the ability of the limb to absorb shock while increasing the flexibility of the iliotibial band. This can be achieved in a number of ways, as outlined below.

Shoes

Injured runners should buy soft running shoes which do not resist pronation. These typically are shoes which have very soft mid-soles, weak heel-counters and are curved and slip-lasted so that they have little resistance to vertical bending around the long axis. In addition, the shoe must not have an outside heel-flare as this has been specifically implicated as an important factor causing this injury. A shoe modification that can be made is to file down the heel flare especially on the outer side but also on the inside of the shoe worn on the injured leg.

In runners with severe bow-legs or very high-arched, rigid feet, it may be necessary for a podiatrist or an orthopaedic technician to build a lateral (outside) wedge into the mid-sole of the shoe. This wedge forces the foot to pronate inwards, thereby improving its shock-absorbing capacity.

Training methods

Athletes should reduce their training, running only to the point of discomfort, never to the point of pain.

Training surfaces

Training should be done on flat, soft surfaces, like grass, and all downhill running must be avoided until the injury has resolved.

Because the majority of ITB injuries occur on the leg furthest away from the centre of the road, all runners should switch the side of the road on which they usually run. (Please note that this advice is potentially dangerous as it is not safe to run with your back to the traffic! Use great caution.)

Stretching

Two special lateral stretches are prescribed. In the first, all the weight is carried on the injured side, and the upper body is bent away from the injured side, with the chest facing forward. This stretches the iliotibial band and should be performed for ten minutes daily (see exercise 14 on page 54). The second stretch is done while sitting. Both hands are placed on the injured knee, which is pulled across the body towards the opposite armpit.

First aid and medical treatment options include icing the tender area of the knee, cross-frictions applied by a physiotherapist to the tender area and hydrocortisone injections into the tender area (but not into the knee joint). Occasionally, in very resistant cases, a small surgical procedure can be performed in which the section of the tendon which comes to ride over the femoral epicondyle is excised. Hydrocortisone injections and surgery should be tried only after all the above treatment options have been tried.

It should be noted that of all running injuries, the success rate in this injury is the most disappointing. While some runners are quickly healed, the ITB friction syndrome can drag on endlessly in others. So if you have to be injured, choose another injury!

The fact that a small percentage of runners who have suffered this injury were ultimately helped when they switched to hard running shoes with prescribed corrective orthotics to limit ankle pronation, suggests that the mechanics causing the injury are not fully understood. Possibly the best advice is to be very cautious with this injury. Rest a lot. When in doubt, rest more.

The Osgood-Schlatter syndrome

Diagnosis

This is a condition specific to growing children who develop discomfort well localized over the tibial tubercle — the knob below the knee cap (see diagram page 110).

Cause

In growing children the tibial tubercle is an epiphysis or a section of bone separated from its shaft by a cartilaginous growth plate. Repetitive contractions by the powerful quadriceps (front of thigh) muscle, which inserts via the patella tendon into the tibial tubercle, can cause minor separation of the epiphyseal cartilage from the underlying bone. The condition resolves when the cartilage in the epiphysis is replaced by bone, usually between fifteen and eighteen years.

Treatment

In the past, immobilization of the knee has been a popular method of treating this condition. But today we know that this is unnecessary and that time alone will cure the injury. Until such time as the tibial epiphysis fuses, the athlete with this condition may continue exercising with discomfort, but not with pain.

Activities that cause pain sufficiently severe to limit exercise must be avoided. Usually this condition occurs in children who participate in a wide variety of sports — for example, rugby, squash and cross-country running. They should cut back a little on all these activities and include more rest days in their schedule. If this fails, they should restrict themselves to one favourite sport.

Chronic muscle tears of the vastus medialis muscles

These are muscles occurring on the front of the thigh immediately above the knee (see diagram page 12). Tearing of these muscles causes pain near the knee.

Diagnosis

The following symptoms indicate the injury:

☐ As with other muscle tears, the onset of pain is gradual and the pain is nagging rather than debilitating.
☐ The pain eases rapidly with rest but recurs with exercise.
☐ Contracting the muscle causes pain. This is done by lying face-up and flexing the knee against resistance. A similar test is done for tears of the quadriceps (see page 106), but of course the site of pain is different.
☐ The injury is tender to the touch and a knot can be felt at the site of pain.

Cause and treatment

These are the same as for the chronic tear of the hamstrings. (See page 102.)

Ismael Kirui *(Kenya)*

Born in Marakwet in Kenya in February 1975. Has been running for as long as he can remember. His primary school was 3 km away and he ran the distance every day in the morning, at lunch time, and in the afternoon. Youngest-ever world track champion, winning the 5000 m in 13:02:75 (a World Junior and Commonwealth record) at 1993 World Championships in Stuttgart, aged eighteen years. In so doing, he defeated top Ethiopian Hailie Gebrselassie by less than a second. Came second in 10 000 m in his first World Junior Championships in 1990 aged fifteen, and fourth in World Junior Cross-Country in same year. Won World Junior Cross-Country title in Boston 1992 and placed third and second respectively in the 1993 and 1995 World Senior Cross-Country Championships. Won the World Cross Challenge Series in 1992–1993. Best times of 7:39:82 and 28:07:1 for 3000 m and 10 000 m respectively. World best 12 km road time of 33:42.

Interview

I received my first injury in 1991. My shins were very painful. It was okay for the first 7 km or so but then it felt like running on hot stone. I had a complete rest for one or two months, and had intensive ultrasound physiotherapy treatment. Because of my patience I was able to enjoy a complete recovery, and my injury has not recurred.

Our comment

The bone injury suffered by Ismael Kirui in 1991 would be expected in a sixteen year old training for, and racing in, international competitions, particularly at the performance levels achieved by this remarkable athlete. Running from an early age will produce bones that are stronger than normal, but it is understandable that even these stronger bones may be unable to cope with the demands of racing in international competition at such an early age.

Rest is the appropriate, indeed the only, treatment for a bone injury. Thereafter the athlete's goal must be to ensure that the injury does not recur.

Aging, because it increases the strength of the bones, naturally reduces the risk of a recurrent injury, as does continued but appropriate training. But excessive training and especially frequent training on an unforgiving synthetic track, will increase the probability that another bone injury will occur. The extent to which Kirui is able to balance the demands he places on his young body will determine whether or not he suffers more injuries of a similar kind.

Popliteus tendonitis

Achilles tendonitis is by far the commonest form of tendonitis. The only other form of this injury that is frequently seen involves the popliteus tendon, which runs around the outside of the knee.

Diagnosis

In this injury there is pain on the outside of the knee just below the site at which the iliotibial band syndrome causes pain (see diagram page 109).

Cause

The injury is said to occur with downhill running although no one has yet studied a large enough number of runners with this injury to confirm this observation. Other causes are probably similar to those for achilles tendonitis and are discussed in more detail under that injury. The most important of these are likely to be increases in training quality (speed) and quantity, and wearing worn-out shoes.

Treatment

The treatment for this injury is the same as that used in the treatment of achilles tendonitis, in particular, the control of ankle pronation with the use of the appropriate shoes and corrective orthotics, and an appropriately reduced training regime in accordance with the seriousness of the injury (grades I to IV).

Lower leg

Posterior and anterior tibial bone strain and fibular bone strain ('shinsplints')

Fifteen years ago, before the running revolution, there was really only one running injury. As long as you were a runner, and you hurt somewhere between the big toes and the hip, then you had 'shinsplints'. Today however, 'shinsplints', which has also been known as medial tibial stress syndrome, is a diagnosis reserved for one specific and curable injury — a bone strain injury localized to one or both of the calf bones (the tibia and the fibula) in one or more of three positions (see diagram page 122).

Tibial and fibular bone strain is the second most common injury, after peripatellar pain syndrome ('runner's knee'), diagnosed in distance runners.

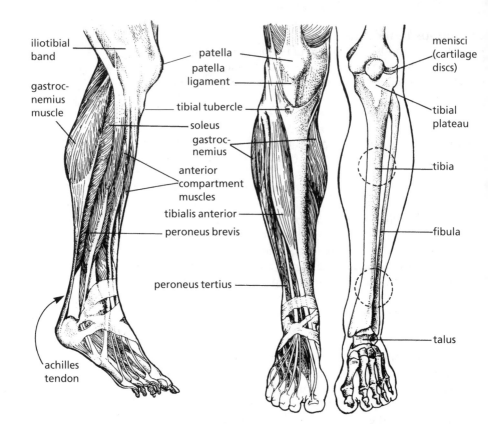

iliotibial band

gastrocnemius muscle

achilles tendon

patella
patella ligament

tibial tubercle

soleus

gastrocnemius

anterior compartment muscles

tibialis anterior

peroneus brevis

peroneus tertius

menisci (cartilage discs)

tibial plateau

tibia

fibula

talus

Diagnosis

Tibial or fibular bone strain typically develops through four stages of injury (second law of running injuries). In the first stage, vague discomfort, poorly localized somewhere in the calf, is noted after exercise. As training continues, the discomfort comes on during exercise. At first it is possible to 'run through' this pain, but if training is continued without treatment, the pain soon becomes so severe that proper training is neither enjoyable nor possible. This is a grade III injury. Ultimately, the injury may be so bad that anything more strenuous than walking is quite impossible. This grade IV bone strain injury has, in fact, become a stress fracture.

In making a diagnosis of bone strain, it is important to differentiate the injury from a chronic tear in the tibialis anterior or tibialis posterior muscles (see diagram above). This is done by feeling for the site at which the greatest tenderness is felt. In bone strain injuries, this is always along either the front (anterior tibial bone strain) or back (posterior tibial bone strain) borders of the tibia or along the outside edge of the fibula (fibular bone strain). These sites are indicated on the diagrams opposite. Usually the bone in the affected area has a rough, corrugated feeling owing to the build-up of a new bony (periosteal) layer at the site of the irritation. When firm finger pressure is applied to these areas, exquisite, well-localized, nauseating tenderness is felt.

Cause

In the 1970s, the most popular explanation was that tibial or fibular bone strain was due to the build-up of pressure in one or more of the tight muscular compartments of the leg during exercise (see diagrams opposite). In true tibial or fibular bone strain, however, there is no such pressure build-up and it appears that 'shinsplints' is a bone injury. Accordingly we prefer to use the term 'bone strain' because there is still confusion among runners as to what 'shinsplints' is. The injury is caused either by excessive ankle pronation or by exposure to excessive shock to which the bone is initially unable to adapt.

The most likely explanation for the majority of cases of tibial or fibular bone strain is that the injury occurs in bones that are undergoing remodelling in response to an increased loading stress. The response of bones to this stress has been discussed under stress fractures (a grade IV bone strain injury) on page 71. Bone strain thus indicates excessive osteoclonal excavation with the development of localized or diffuse areas of bone weakness. These weaker areas are sensitive to touch, as well as to the increased loading stress of exercise.

Three mechanisms appear to be the main contributors to this injury. These are overstriding, excessive ankle pronation and poor shock-absorption.

Overstriding is thought to be the major cause of anterior tibial bone strain. Overstriding causes the forefoot to slap onto the ground and it is believed that in trying to prevent this slapping movement, the muscles in the front of the calf are forced to overwork. Ultimately pain develops at the point where they attach to the tibia.

Posterior tibial bone strain, by far the most common form of bone strain, is almost certainly caused by either excessive ankle pronation or the inadequate shock-absorbing ability of bones not used to the stresses of running. It is probable that abnormal ankle pronation causes a twisting force to develop in the tibia and the fibula and that this eventually leads to minute bone cracks at the sites of greatest bone resorption, causing the pain. (These minute bone cracks could be grade I to IV injuries.)

Tibial and fibular bone strain is most common among five groups of athletes: middle-distance high school track athletes, beginning joggers, competitive female runners, female aerobic dancers (especially instructors) and army recruits during their first few months of training. The more experienced runners are susceptible when they start training intensively for competition. Other factors associated with the injury are as follows:

Training errors, training surfaces and running shoes

The typical training routine of the high school track athlete provides a perfect recipe for bone strain. Little training is done in the off-season, so that when the new season begins the athlete is exposed to an impossible training load. This usually takes the form of too much speedwork, too often, too soon, with no hard day/easy day routine. This is done under the worst possible environmental conditions of running continually in one direction on a hard unforgiving running surface, in hard uncompromising shoes. Unless the athlete has perfect lower limbs and very strong bones, the end result of bone strain or a stress fracture is predictable.

Beginner or experienced distance runners who subject themselves to similar training errors of too much, too fast, too soon and wear inappropriate shoes (see shoes page 36) expose themselves to similar risks.

Hereditary factors

These are essentially the same as those causing peripatellar pain syndrome — in particular, hypermobile feet which pronate excessively and a leg-length discrepancy. In addition, there may be inadequate flexibility of the ankle caused by tight calf muscles. It is also possible that some runners may have bones that are genetically weak. This will automatically put them at risk.

Muscle imbalance and inflexibility

It is believed that the strength of the posterior calf muscles is increased more by running than the strength of the anterior (front) calf muscles. This strength imbalance may then play a role in bone strain injury.

Weak bones caused by menstrual abnormalities or a low-calcium diet or both

Depressed blood levels of the female hormone oestrogen and low dietary calcium intake in women runners who have menstrual abnormalities weaken their bones and expose them to a higher incidence of bone injuries. That bones weakened by these factors are more prone to injury was first shown by UCT Sports Science graduate and former Springbok gymnast, Dr Kathy Myburgh. These factors are further discussed under stress fractures on page 74.

Treatment

Successful treatment of tibial and fibular bone strain should aim to address the cause of the injury. Once one or more of the factors outlined above have been identified as contributing to the injury, these can be addressed in an effective treatment programme.

For grade I injuries which cause pain only after exercise the first priority is to determine whether anything has changed recently in the runner's training methods. A return to previous training methods or the purchase of appropriate running shoes may be all that is required to cure the injury. If the runner pronates excessively, a strong anti-pronation shoe is required. If not, a softer shoe may be needed to absorb shock more effectively.

Novice runners who have been running for under three months can be reassured that it is likely that their injury will disappear in four to ten weeks without any specific treatment, and even without a reduction in training. This recovery will indicate that their bones have strengthened and adapted to the increased load. Attention must be paid to the running gait: in particular, injured runners must learn to run with a shuffle and to avoid overstriding. Another trick is to avoid pushing off with the toes, which should rather be allowed to float inside the shoe.

Another treatment option, where tight calf muscles and/or muscle imbalance have been identified, is to do specific calf-muscle stretching and strengthening exercises. Appropriate exercises are shown on pages 51 and 52 (7 and 10).

A specific form of treatment that can be used in all cases of bone strain is to apply ice massages to the sore areas for twenty to thirty minutes a session, two to three times a day. The ice should be placed in a plastic container and then massaged gently up and down the leg over the sore areas.

Women who are not menstruating regularly should, if they are knowingly restricting their food intakes, consider increasing their food intakes until normal menstrual patterns return. Alternatively they should consult a gynaecologist for an opinion about the advisability of taking replacement oestrogen and progesterone therapy.

Women who are restricting their dietary calcium intakes, usually by avoiding dairy products which provide most of the calcium in the diet, should consider taking supplementary calcium in the form of calcium tablets (500–1000 mg per day).

When, despite trying everything listed above, pain is always present during running (grade II and III injuries), the only real hope for a cure is to acquire a corrective orthotic to wear when running. Only when the orthotic is correctly adjusted, however, will it cure the injury. If the corrective orthotic fails to provide a cure, it is likely it has not been made sufficiently well to provide the precise degree of control required to cure the injury.

Stress fracture of the tibia

The tibia or shin bone is the most vulnerable of all bones to stress fractures in distance runners, accounting for more than half the total number of stress fractures.

The commonest sites for tibial stress fractures are immediately below the tibial plateau, 5 cm below the knee or at the junction of the lower third and upper two thirds of the tibia (see diagram page 122). The fracture 5 cm below the knee is especially common in novice runners.

The diagnosis, cause and treatment of these stress fractures are as described in the general discussion on stress fractures on page 68, but the salient features are listed here for convenience.

Diagnosis

☐ The injury occurs suddenly with no external violence involved.

☐ Hopping on the injured leg is painful. Running is impossible.

☐ Extreme tenderness is felt, localized to the bone at one or more of the sites mentioned above.

☐ The injury heals completely within two to three months of complete rest.

Cause

Training errors in the form of sudden increases in training load through longer distances, more speed and frequent racing, or a heavy training load for many months, appear to be the major problem. The bone is subjected to increased load before it is ready to cope with it. Novices are particularly vulnerable, as are women with abnormal menstruation.

Treatment

The only recognized treatment is complete rest from running for eight to twelve weeks. Runners may obtain relief from their symptoms for this stress fracture by wearing a pneumatic leg brace and there is some evidence that exposing the injury to an electric field or exercising in water may speed the healing process.

The stress fracture of the anterior border of the tibia (felt as a sharp ridge down the centre front of the leg) is an uncommon injury and should be diagnosed and treated in the same way as above.

Stress fracture of the fibula

Although the fibula or small calf bone (see diagram on page 122) is not a major weight-bearing bone, its thin structure and its propensity to sideways movement under load make it vulnerable to stress fractures. It has been estimated that the fibula accounts for fourteen percent of all stress fractures. The fibula is also prone to fracture during a severe ankle sprain. The diagnosis, cause and treatment of this fracture is similar to what is described on page 126. The specific features of the fibula fracture are highlighted here.

Diagnosis

Diagnosis is sometimes difficult as the pain does not always prevent running completely as virtually all other stress fractures do. In addition, the pain may be difficult to localize. The clearest diagnosis is tenderness localized over the fibula. When this sign is present and the athlete is unable to run, the diagnosis is a fibular stress fracture.

A more common cause of fracture of the fibula is severe ankle sprain. Bruising extends up the side of the leg and the fibula is sore to the touch. As this is not a stress fracture, but rather the result of external trauma, an X-ray is required. If a fracture is shown on the X-ray, it must be treated appropriately by an orthopaedic surgeon. Do not try to run for four to six weeks.

Bruce Fordyce (see page 17)

Interview

I'm a strong pronator and my muscle injuries have been related to over-pronation in training. I first had a problem in 1980 when a torn quadriceps kept me from training much in February in my build-up to the Comrades.

Then in 1982, again in February, I tore my soleus [calf] muscles in both legs. That worried me at first because I could not get rid of the injuries and they were really painful. I thought I had stress fractures, but then they were correctly identified as calf tears. Once the injury and its cause had been accurately diagnosed I was soon cured. I received cross-friction physiotherapy and changed my shoes and had no more problems.

Actually, it was these injuries which led me to realize that I did not need to train hard in February to do well in the Comrades. In 1980 I was concerned about this apparent gaping hole in my programme preparation, but I had a good run anyway. My 1982 injury confirmed what I had already suspected, that one's hard training for Comrades should begin only in March. [Fordyce placed second in the 87 km race in 1980, two minutes behind Alan Robb. In 1982 he won the race for the second year in succession.]

As I enter my forties, I find that I have to be even more tuned in to my body to avoid injury. My soleus still threatens to tear now and then. Fortunately I know myself well enough to spot the warning signs and either change to a more supportive shoe or rest to avoid falling victim to the injury.

In general I train a bit less than I used to. I take that much longer to recover from a quality session than before and I'm also markedly stiffer than I used to be. This has led to some hamstring problems. It is vital for me to identify an injury as early as possible to prevent it from becoming significant.

I should counter these problems by regular stretching, but I tend to be lazy about this aspect.

Our comment

It is perhaps only in retrospect that Bruce Fordyce's true brilliance as an ultra-marathon runner has been appreciated.

The measure of his genius was not that he ran the Comrades Marathon faster than any athlete in the history of the race, but that he ran well so frequently (nine wins, preceded by a third and second position). The key to his longevity at the top seems to have been an exceptional capacity to recover from the muscle damage of each year's race. This must have been the result of his diligent approach to training, his astute ability to monitor his body, and a unique genetic gift.

Fordyce's intelligent methods, even more apparent in his approach to his now-aging body, remain the gold-standard for all who wish to emulate his achievements in any athletic event.

Cause
Biomechanical factors at present unknown cause a concentration of stress in the fibula. It has been suggested that excessive sideways pull by the leg muscles on the fibula during repetitive action, such as running, leads to stress fractures in the fibula. As is the case with other fractures, these are also associated with sudden changes in training activity, such as increasing too rapidly the total distance or amount of speedwork incorporated in a training programme. Increased training will often lead to muscle tightness which could increase the sideways pull on the bone.

Bones weakened by the factors already described are more likely to fracture.

Treatment
The only effective treatment is complete rest from running. The injury should heal within four to six weeks. If it takes longer to heal, consider the possibility that the fracture occurred in an area of bone weakened by, for example, a bone cyst or some other abnormality unrelated to running. Under these circumstances, an X-ray becomes essential.

Chronic tears of the calf muscles
The calf musculature consists mainly of two muscles — the gastrocnemius, the prominent muscle of the upper calf, and the soleus, the muscle of the lower calf (see diagram page 122).

The diagnosis, cause and treatment of these injuries is essentially the same as what is described in the section on chronic muscle tears in general on page 80, but the salient points are listed here for convenience.

Diagnosis

Discomfort is localized to the calf muscles. When the pain develops, the athlete is unable to push off strongly with the ankle on the affected side. Rising on tiptoe may reproduce the pain. The onset of pain is gradual but interferes with training (especially speedwork) if left untreated. The pain passes quickly with rest but is not cured unless vigorous cross-frictions are given.

Cause

An unaccustomed amount of calf muscle activity through excessive speedwork induces muscle fatigue and makes muscles vulnerable to tears. Muscles tear during eccentric contraction and may therefore be undertrained for eccentric muscle contractions. Collapsed shoe mid-soles appear to exacerbate the problem.

Treatment

The only effective treatment is a series of cross-friction applications to the torn site. Ultrasound after the cross-frictions may be of help. Training with eccentric muscle contractions (walking and running backwards downhill) may make it less likely that the injury will recur.

Chronic tears of the muscles alongside the shin bone

Diagnosis

Chronic muscle tears of the anterior or posterior tibial muscles (see diagram page 122) cause the greatest pain to be felt in the muscle, as distinct from bone strain and stress fractures, which cause the most pain to be felt on the bone. The muscles will be exquisitely tender at the injured site, where a 'knot' will be felt. In the case of the posterior tibial muscle the tender site may be very deep-seated, under the main calf muscle. Pain will be felt by contracting the muscle against resistance. In the case of the anterior muscle this is achieved by attempting to pull the toes of the injured leg towards you. Flex the ankle against resistance provided by pushing down on the toes with the other foot. In the case of the posterior muscle the foot and toes should be pushed down hard against a resistance, simultaneously turning the foot inwards.

Cause

The anterior tibial muscle tear is more often caused by an external force, such as tripping while running, than by overuse. The reverse is true of the posterior muscle tear, although this can arise as a result of a severe ankle sprain. Modification of training methods or surfaces and worn-out shoes have been identified as important contributors to the latter injury. The posterior muscle in particular can be torn by excessive ankle pronation. Other causes are discussed in the section on chronic muscle tears on page 80.

Treatment

As discussed on page 82, the primary treatment must be a series of cross-friction treatments, although there is some indication that regular icing and gentle stretching may also be of help. Corrective orthotics should be used by those who pronate excessively.

Delayed muscle soreness of the calf muscles

This occurs in people who are undertrained or who race a long distance, such as a marathon. The injury is exacerbated by a tendency to run on the toes, which increases the eccentric loading of the calf muscles. To compensate for the consequent tightening of the muscles, adequate stretching of the calf muscles should be carried out before and after exercise (see 7 and 10 on pages 51 and 52). Eccentric muscle training (running or walking downhill backwards) may reduce the likelihood of a recurrence. This injury is fully discussed on page 77.

Cramping of the calf muscles

Muscle cramps are discussed in detail on page 84.

Chronic compartment syndrome

In the compartment syndromes, exercise causes an abnormal rise in pressure in one or more of the muscular compartments of the lower leg (see diagram page 122).

Diagnosis

The most common symptom in the chronic form of this injury is the onset of pain during or after exercise. At first, the pain is mild and disappears rapidly as soon as the runner stops running. However, with time, the pain becomes progressively more severe and begins to interfere with running. Ultimately the pain is so severe that it forces the patient to stop running.

The site of pain is well localized — it usually occurs in the deep posterior calf muscles, less commonly in the anterior and lateral calf muscles (see diagram page 122). The distinctive feature characterizing this injury is that as the affected muscles become painful, they lose their normal suppleness and become very hard to the touch. In fact, they become rock hard. But as the pain disappears, so the hardness gradually dissipates.

Differentiating compartment syndromes from tibial or fibular bone strain

The ratio of runners suffering from true tibial or fibular bone strain to those with the compartment syndrome is of the order of 100:1 to 200:1. This indicates just how uncommon this injury is. A true compartment syndrome can be differentiated from bone strain with relative ease because:

☐ it causes pain localized to the muscles, not to the bones, of the lower limb;
☐ the injury never gets better even after months of rest (whereas in bone strain the runner will usually be pain-free after a few months' rest);
☐ after running, the involved muscles become absolutely rock hard and the foot may be pulled into a strange position (because of transient muscle paralysis);
☐ muscle weakness and even muscle paralysis may develop;
☐ there may also be changes in skin sensation and occasionally, severe muscle cramping: the runner usually complains that the foot 'goes numb'.

Cause

In people who develop this injury, the muscle compartments do not allow sufficient room for normal muscle swelling during exercise. The resultant pressure increase may be so great that it obstructs the blood flow to the muscles, causing them to become painful.

At present, the only factors known to be associated with this injury are hereditary — muscle compartments that are too small to accommodate the normal swelling of the muscles they contain during exercise, or muscles that are simply too big for their compartments.

Treatment

There is only one type of treatment for this injury and that is a surgical procedure in which the lining of the tight compartment is split, allowing the muscle to expand freely inside its compartment. Rest and other forms of conservative treatment are almost always unsuccessful. It is important that all the involved compartments are identified and surgically treated. The deep posterior compartment in particular needs to be released. However, involvement of this compartment is the most difficult to diagnose.

The response to treatment is excellent if the initial diagnosis was correct; the athlete is again able to run pain-free as soon as the surgical wound has healed. If the condition does not resolve with surgery, it is usually because the deep posterior compartment is also involved and was not released during surgery.

Acute compartment syndrome

Diagnosis

When acute compartment syndrome sets in, the athlete has had no previous warning of impending disaster. Suddenly the muscles become progressively more painful after a single exercise session.

Usually this occurs in relatively untrained runners, especially army recruits after a single very severe bout of exercise. Instead of abating with rest, the pain intensifies dramatically. The runner may also notice loss of sensation in the skin overlying the muscles, and ultimately there may be paralysis of those muscles which also become board-hard. By this stage, arterial pulses in the foot will have disappeared.

Cause

The pressure inside the compartment suddenly builds up to such an extent that it interferes with blood flow to the involved muscles. As these muscles have an inadequate blood supply they first become painful. If the pressure is not relieved and adequate blood flow restored, the muscles will be irrevocably damaged and will die.

Treatment

The treatment is to relieve the pressure without delay. This is achieved by the same surgical procedure used in the management of the more insidious (chronic) form of compartment syndrome. The only difference is that for this acute form of the injury, the surgery must be performed as an absolute emergency, as soon as it becomes clear that the pain will not subside.

Achilles tendonitis

Achilles tendonitis is one of the most debilitating injuries and has curtailed the training programmes and modified the aspirations of many great and not-so-great runners. It ranks third behind peripatellar pain syndrome and bone strain in terms of frequency of occurrence in runners. It becomes increasingly common in older athletes.

Diagnosis

Unlike muscle injuries, which are usually poorly recognized by runners and their advisers, tendon injuries do not usually present a diagnostic problem to anyone, particularly when they occur, as they usually do, in the achilles tendon.

The first inkling of disaster usually comes with the first step out of bed in the morning. As soon as the afflicted foot touches the ground there is a feeling of discomfort or stiffness behind the ankle. This is usually enough to cause some initial limping which tends to wear off after a few minutes of walking. These symptoms constitute a grade I injury. If the condition is allowed to progress unchecked, discomfort may also be noted after exercise, particularly after long runs or fast intervals (grade II) and this may deteriorate gradually through grades III and IV of injury (second law of running injuries).

As has already been stated, the diagnosis of achilles tendonitis is usually very easy. The discomfort is localized to the tendon and on pinching the tendon between the thumb and index finger, one or more exquisitely tender areas are located.

Cause

The most probable cause of achilles tendonitis is that excessive ankle pronation causes a whipping action or bowstring effect in the achilles tendon. The achilles tendon has a relatively poor blood supply in the area in which it typically develops the injury — that is, 2 cm to 6 cm above the site of insertion of the tendon into the heel bone. It is likely that this whipping action interferes with the already tenuous blood supply to the area, leading ultimately to the death of small areas of the tendon in that region. Alternatively, a more modern explanation is that

Elana Meyer

(see page 25)

Interview   *I had a hard few months of racing between July and August
1989 and in hindsight I don't feel I gave my body enough time
to recover. I kept on pushing to get back into training for the
next event and I suppose something had to give.*

*I had raced the SA National Half-Marathon Championships
[69:26 — fourth fastest in the world], the SA National Cross-
Country Championships, the Prestige Cross-Country, the Cape
Town Street Mile, the Momentum Life 15 km and the Champion
of Champions event within ten weeks, many on consecutive
weekends. [With the exception of the half-marathon, in which
she placed second, Meyer won each of these events against the
toughest opposition in the country.]*

*During the week after the Champion of Champions event
[comprising three 10 km races on track, cross-country and road
within five days] both my achilles tendons became painful while
I was training. I was eventually forced to rest.*

*I received the usual treatment — lots of ice and physiotherapy.
I did no running at all in the two weeks before the national 15 km
championships in early November, but decided to risk giving it a
go anyway. However, my achilles felt sore from the start and
after only 6 km I was simply forced to stop.*

*After another month of treatment I was able to resume train-
ing in December, but it was only in April 1990 that I was completely free from pain.*

*I have had to learn to live with the injury and my approach
since 1993 is to prevent a recurrence of the injury, rather than
wait for it to happen and then treat it. By going to physiotherapy three to four times a week I have been able to keep it in
check and fortunately my training or racing programme has not
been significantly affected in recent years.*

Our comment   Achilles tendon injuries tend to recur, especially in elite athletes
who must maintain their speed and who cannot therefore
afford not to race and train relatively frequently at high
intensity. 'Preventative maintenance' as practised by Meyer is
therefore the only solution for the injured, elite athlete who
wishes to sustain a career at the top of the sport.

the achilles tendon is an important shock-absorbing structure and that age and minor injury reduce its ability to absorb shock. Excessive loading, especially eccentric loading, then promotes further injury. There may be a number of risk factors for this injury:

Training factors

The injury can be brought on by any sudden increase in training distances, in particular single, very long runs; too many speed sessions, particularly if these are done by running mainly on the toes; a sudden return to heavy training after lay-off; and increased inflexibility of the calf muscles caused by too much training and too little stretching. Also see training methods on page 30.

Shoes

Problems can be caused by shoes that

- [ ] are heelless spikes or low-heeled shoes (racing flats);
- [ ] are worn out;
- [ ] are inappropriate to the individual runner's specific biomechanical needs;
- [ ] have a heel height of under 12 mm to 15 mm;
- [ ] have a very stiff sole that fails to bend easily at the forefoot;
- [ ] are excessively hard and therefore increase the loading of the tendon.

Wearing high heels at work during the day promotes calf-muscle shortening so that when the runner changes to lower-heeled running shoes, the achilles tendon is suddenly put on the stretch. The only time it is a good idea to wear high-heeled shoes, is during the early treatment phase of this injury. Also see shoe selection on page 36.

Genetic factors

These include tight, inflexible calf muscles, hypermobile feet, and in a small percentage of runners, the high-arched, cavus or 'clunk' foot. Possibly there are genetic differences in the ability of different tendons to absorb shock.

Other factors

Age and many years of heavy training seem also to make this injury more likely. Older runners who try to train as they did in their youth appear to be at risk.

Treatment

Ice
The initial treatment for the injured achilles tendon is to apply an ice-pack to the sore area for as long as is possible, each day. A suggested schedule is to apply an ice pack for at least thirty minutes, three times a day, especially immediately before and after running.

Stretching
Appropriate calf-muscle stretching exercises must be done for between ten and twenty minutes each day. The most effective stretching exercises are 7 and 10 on pages 51 and 52.

In addition, eccentric stretching of the achilles tendon (to allow the tendon to be loaded in a stretched position) may be very helpful. This would increase the strength of the achilles tendon during eccentric loading (such as running downhill).

Drugs
Although anti-inflammatory drugs and/or cortisone injections are often prescribed, they have several disadvantages:

☐ This treatment could suggest that a cure can be bought or swallowed. Only by learning why the injury happened will a runner ever learn how to avoid further injury.
☐ The money could, perhaps, be better spent on a new pair of shoes, which might have more lasting curative effects. The same could be said of this book!
☐ There is a risk that cortisone injected into the tendon may make it more liable to rupture completely. In fact, it is very hard to condone giving a cortisone injection into the achilles tendon. It implies buying a short-term benefit at a massive long-term cost — the risk of tendon rupture requiring emergency surgery.

Shoes
When choosing a shoe to treat achilles tendonitis, look for anti-pronation models with rigid heel-counters and firmer mid-sole material that best reduce excessive ankle pronation. However, such shoes must still offer reasonable shock absorption.

A 7 mm to 15 mm heel raise should be added to the running shoes, either as an addition to the heel, or as firm felt material inside the running shoe. This is especially important in people who have either tight calf muscles, cavus (high-arched) feet, or leg-length inequalities.

If the achilles tendonitis resists all the above treatment, then a corrective orthotic is indicated, particularly for the excessive pronator. These should be professionally made and will usually require expert readjustment before they are completely effective. Also see page 39.

Rest or modification of training schedule
It may be that an attack of achilles tendonitis is an indication for total rest until the injury has healed. The injury can cause scarring between the achilles tendon and its sheath which could be aggravated by continued running.

But as few runners will even consider this advice, a more acceptable approach is one of modified rest tailored to the grade of injury. An outline of such a training programme is given on page 33.

One way of tailoring training to the injury is to use the 'pinch test' after each run. If the test indicates that the tendon is becoming progressively more tender after a particular training session, then this indicates either that total training should be reduced, or that that particular training session should be avoided. Alternatively, if the tendon becomes progressively less tender, then the treatment is succeeding and training distance and intensity may be gradually increased.

Physiotherapy
This is advised for all injuries and should be mandatory for all injuries worse than grade I. The most effective type of physio-therapy is vigorous cross-frictions applied to the tender areas of the tendon. This should be followed by ultrasound treatment.

Surgery
The ultimate danger in recurrent achilles tendonitis is that the scarring process, which initially starts inside the tendon, progresses to involve the sheath surrounding the tendon. When this happens, adhesions (connections) are formed between the tendon and its sheath. As this happens, the free movement of the tendon inside its sheath becomes increasingly impaired and the tendon becomes susceptible to repeated attacks of tendonitis. Each of these leaves the runner progressively more debilitated until ultimately very little running is possible.

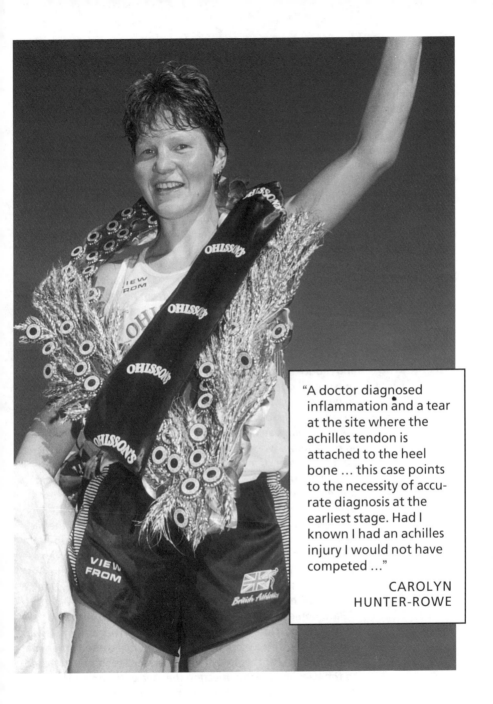

"A doctor diagnosed inflammation and a tear at the site where the achilles tendon is attached to the heel bone ... this case points to the necessity of accurate diagnosis at the earliest stage. Had I known I had an achilles injury I would not have competed ..."

CAROLYN HUNTER-ROWE

Carolyn Hunter-Rowe (United Kingdom)

Began running competitively in 1989 aged twenty-five. Immediate interest in ultra-distance events and won London to Brighton 88 km in 7:18:09 just two years later. Placed third at the World 100 km Championships in Spain in 1992 before winning the British 100 km Championships in the Commonwealth record of 7:39:59. Set World track records over 25 miles, 30 miles and 50 km in 1992, and improved them a year later, setting a 50 km time of 3:26:43. In 1993 won World 100 km title in Belgium in Commonwealth record time of 7:27:19, won London to Brighton 55 miler in 6:34:10 (course record), and won the Langburgh Marathon in the course record of 2:44:32. Named *Runner's World* Best Female Distance Runner of 1993. Won 1994 Malta Marathon in a PB of 2:40:28 (course record) and the Two Oceans 56 km Marathon in Cape Town two months later; set her 10 km best of 35:19 in 1994.

Interview

I generally plan my training and racing programme carefully, giving me sufficient time to recover from racing. Although my training mileage is high, I always incorporate one rest day per week. I stretch regularly, about fifteen to twenty minutes each day. If I miss out on stretching, I immediately notice the difference in my muscle tightness. If I have a slight niggle I am careful and reduce my training. If I cannot explain it, I take off a day or two until it goes away. I make sure I eat very well. I've tried not to be preoccupied with losing weight, but concentrate on eating healthy foods.

About four weeks before the 1994 World 100 km Championships in Japan, where I was defending my title, I began to feel a pain at the rear of my heel. It was diagnosed as a heel bursitis and I had physiotherapy treatment in the form of ultrasound and electrowave treatment. In addition, I iced my heel after every run and took a course of anti-inflammatories.

The pain eased slightly, but worsened in the week of the race. Believing the problem to be a bursa, I thought I could run through the injury. During the race I began to have problems after 10 km which I kept at bay until 70 km. Running the race was the most painful experience of my life but (foolishly) I felt I had to finish for the team event.

Back home I had to wait three weeks before I could get a specialist's opinion, during which I did only cross training (swimming, cycling and weights). Then a doctor diagnosed inflammation and a tear at the site where the achilles tendon is attached to the heel bone. After injecting the area with cortisone and resting for a further week I started running again.

To me this case points to the necessity of an accurate diagnosis at the earliest stage. Had I known that I had an achilles injury, I would not have competed in Japan. In addition, it taught me never to start an ultra-distance race with an injury.

Our comment   Achilles tendon injuries heal slowly and often incompletely, so they frequently recur. Recurrent achilles tendon injuries are often the reason why athletes must terminate their competitive careers. Hunter-Rowe has learned that when the achilles tendon hurts, the best treatment is to stop running and seek appropriate medical advice. Running should only commence when there is no pain in the tendon when running.

Fortunately, this injury can now be very effectively treated by a delicate surgical procedure which removes the tendon sheath together with any areas of tendon scarring. When performed by an experienced surgeon, this procedure has been shown to have a very high success rate. However, surgery should be considered only when all other techniques, including repeated sessions of vigorous cross-frictions, have been without effect.

Partial or complete tear of the achilles tendon

Diagnosis
Two serious conditions involving the achilles tendon, need to be differentiated from achilles tendonitis. In the partial or complete tendon ruptures, either a large portion of the tendon (partial) or the complete tendon ruptures, causing sudden dramatic pain and weakness in the affected leg. Although complete achilles tendon rupture is an uncommon injury in distance runners, the incomplete tear is not infrequently seen, as described by Ewald Bonzet on page 142.

The importance of recognizing complete or partial achilles tendon ruptures is that they are conditions for which early surgery may be essential. Thus if the onset of achilles tendon pain is sudden and debilitating, unlike the gradual onset described for typical achilles tendonitis, then it is essential that the runner seek out an experienced surgeon without delay. This must be done so that the appropriate surgery can be performed urgently. The area of torn tendon begins to degenerate shortly

Ewald Bonzet *(South Africa)*

One of the most versatile SA athletes of all time, with top performances in all distances between the mile (3:57) and the marathon (2:12:08). Earned national colours in track, cross-country, and road running. Won SA titles at senior level at cross-country (1979), track (10 000 m in 1982), and on the road (16 km in 1981 and the marathon in 1983). Ran 2:12:08 in his debut marathon at Stellenbosch in 1983, but failed to improve on the time.

Won 1983 interprovincial marathon title in Port Elizabeth in gale-force winds in 2:13:54. Ran 2:17 at the Chicago Marathon in 1984 after running at 2:07 pace (with de Castella, Jones and Lopes) for 20 miles, but slowed over final 6 miles. Still competitive as a veteran runner. Is held in considerable esteem as a coach, as indicated by the fact that Elana Meyer appointed him as her coach in September 1995.

Interview

I'd been having achilles problems intermittently for which I'd had cortisone injections. I had such an injection shortly before the SA National Cross-Country Championships in Port Elizabeth in 1987. I was leading the sub-veterans race over 10 km when it happened. A number of 'speedbumps' had been placed on the course. I landed toe-first on one of them, in full stride, and at that moment I felt my achilles go. The pain was debilitating. I should have stopped immediately but tried to continue and that was where it tore again. My leg was black and blue all over — it was incredible.

On the basis of the fact that it had not torn away completely I decided to risk not having surgery, but it took nineteen months before I could run comfortably again. Initially I could barely walk — I was a complete cripple! Fortunately I have made a hundred percent recovery, thus vindicating my decision to avoid surgery. Because of scar tissue, though, my right achilles is about twice as thick as my left, but the main thing is that I can run without pain.

One of the major problems with one's achilles is that during the day we wear shoes with a higher heel and then we go out to train in flat running shoes. Regular stretching is essential to avoid the problem.

Our comment Clinical trials indicate that surgery and immobilization are equally valuable in the management of acute tears of the achilles tendon. But whichever treatment is chosen, it must be initiated early. If immobilization is chosen, this must be secure.

Especially in the case of a complete tear of the achilles tendon, any movement at the site of the tear will produce a less than ideal result and may leave the tendon weakened. Bonzet's recovery seems to have taken a longer time than might normally have been expected, perhaps because his injured tendon may not have been adequately immobilized early in treatment. But the fact that he continues to run competitively is the more important measure of the success of the treatment method used.

Achilles tendon injuries are probably the most common reason why elite athletes, like Bonzet, who have been successful on the track for decades, eventually have to retire. Former world mile record holders, New Zealander John Walker and Irishman Eammon Coghlan, were both forced to terminate their track racing careers in the early forties because of chronic achilles tendon injuries which prevented the speed training necessary to remain competitive in track competition.

---

after injury, making surgery extremely difficult after any delay.

In a completely ruptured (and a severe partially ruptured) tendon it should be possible to feel a complete gap in the tendon. An important feature of a complete tendon rupture is that it prevents normal walking on the affected side. The runner with a completely ruptured achilles tendon is unable to push off with that ankle, because the calf muscles that provide the power for push-off are no longer attached to the ankle by the achilles tendon.

Cause

The cause of the complete or partial tear is essentially similar to that described for achilles tendonitis above. The partial or complete tear often occurs after a normal case of tendonitis has been aggravated, possibly by the intensification of some of the factors previously described or following a cortisone injection. If the tendon has already been weakened in some way it is more likely to tear. As was the case with Ewald Bonzet's rupture, the tendon usually tears during eccentric loading. This indicates that it is the loss of eccentric strength that predisposes to this injury. Age is an important factor that makes this injury more likely.

Treatment

Immediate surgery by a skilled orthopaedic surgeon is indicated for the partial or complete tear of the achilles tendon. Although there are some grounds for arguing a more conservative approach to the treatment of partial tears, it is probable that such an approach is likely to delay the return of the athlete to competitive running longer than if surgery had been performed. This could leave the tendon in a weaker state through the accumulation of scar tissue. In other words, the likelihood of a good result is reduced if surgery is not performed.

Popliteal artery entrapment syndrome

Diagnosis

This is an extremely uncommon injury that causes pain in the leg during exercise. The symptoms may suggest either a compartment syndrome or a chronic muscle tear. Differentiation from these more common injuries is for the experts only, and the injury should be referred to them when it fails to respond to treatment for these injuries, or when its symptoms fail to correspond with those of the conventional injuries.

Cause

The injury is caused by the contraction of an accessory portion of the gastrocnemius muscle (see diagram page 122) that surrounds the main artery in the calf, the popliteal artery. Contraction of that muscle during exercise causes obstruction of the artery, preventing adequate blood flow to the calf. It is this absence of blood flow that causes the pain during exercise.

Treatment

The only effective treatment is surgery by an experienced vascular surgeon. Occasionally the artery is damaged and needs to be repaired.

Effort thrombosis of the deep calf veins

Effort thrombosis (clotting of the blood) of the deep calf veins is a very uncommon injury. The injury, which can be precipitated by exercise, is, however, extremely dangerous. The main danger of this condition is that a part of the blood clot can dislodge and travel through the heart to lodge in the arteries of the lungs. If sufficiently large, the dislodged clot can cause death within minutes; if smaller, it causes the death of small areas of the lung. When this occurs the patient will experience marked chest pain and may cough up blood.

Diagnosis
Once the clot has formed it blocks the main route for blood to return from the legs to the heart. The blood then accumulates in the legs, causing pain, especially in the calf. The pain may subside after exercise but will recur once running is resumed. Later, as the extent of the clot increases, the ankle and calf will begin to swell.

Cause
The factors precipitating the clotting are unknown. The condition is so uncommon that some hereditary predisposition or some associated medical condition must be at work.

Treatment
The only treatment is immediate hospitalization to allow for the safe administration of drugs that reduce blood clotting; supportive bandaging of the leg; and a complete avoidance of all exercise for a period of up to six to twelve months. During this period, blood clotting is controlled with appropriate medication. Fortunately, recovery is usually complete.

Ankle

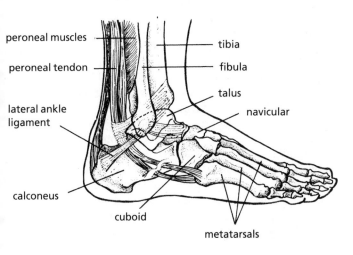

peroneal muscles

tibia

peroneal tendon

fibula

talus

lateral ankle ligament

navicular

calconeus

cuboid

metatarsals

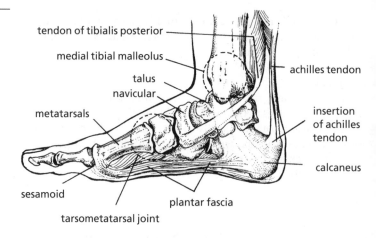

tendon of tibialis posterior
medial tibial malleolus
talus
navicular
metatarsals
sesamoid
tarsometatarsal joint
plantar fascia
achilles tendon
insertion of achilles tendon
calcaneus

Inversion strain

Sprained ankles do not fall into the category of intrinsic injuries, but are injuries often incurred by runners, especially those running over uneven terrain, such as in cross-country competition. At best they cause mild local pain and may require a couple of days' rest from training. At worst they can be absolutely debilitating, requiring surgical correction of the damaged ligaments and bones.

Diagnosis

In the case of inversion strain (also known as lateral ligament strain) there will be localized pain and swelling. The injury may be painful at rest or after taking a few steps. Pain is produced when the heel bone is moved inwards or if the big toe is pointed downwards and inwards.

Where rupture of the lateral (outside) ligaments has occurred, the pain will be excruciating and significant swelling will take place around the joint. The ankle joint will have become destabilized, with the talus, the main ankle bone, having been released from its ligament clamp and able to move too freely.

Depending on the severity of the injury, a spiral fracture of the fibula could occur as much as 15 cm above its lower end. Bruising and swelling above the ankle and tenderness over the bone are diagnostic of this complication. Fractures of the tips of the fibula and tibia (the fibular and tibial malleoli) could be an additional complication in severe cases. An X-ray is necessary to exclude these complications.

Cause

This injury is caused simply by turning the ankle over onto the outside of the foot in one way or another. This forces the ankle into an abnormal position.

Treatment

The rapidity with which the athlete is able to walk normally after injury is a useful indicator of the severity of the injury. A mild sprain which will need relatively little treatment will allow the runner to run fairly normally within a few minutes. This injury can be treated at home according to the principles set out below.

Symptoms that persist for any longer require that the athlete consult an orthopaedic surgeon or, at the very least, have a thorough radiological evaluation of the ankle performed.

The well-established ICE treatment should be used as a first aid measure. ICE stands for ice, compression and elevation. Frequent applications of ice or a cold pack should be used, especially on the first day. The ankle should be kept at an elevation above the hip for as long as possible to reduce swelling. Support bandaging should be used (either the air cast, pneumatic splint or stirrup strap) to maintain the ankle in the normal position.

Cross-friction followed by ultrasound should be applied where there is ligament damage and strengthening exercises should be prescribed to re-establish full use of the ankle. Working the injured muscles against a force provided by anchored rubber tubing will be effective. In addition, it is important to restore the balance mechanisms which operate through the ankle. This can be done by progressively more difficult balancing exercises, balancing on one leg with closed eyes. Return to running with caution, never running to the point of pain. Maintain strapping on runs until six weeks after the pain has passed.

This rehabilitation process must be under the care of a trained specialist, especially a physiotherapist.

When the injury is less severe, the injured athlete can run again almost immediately, provided that the supporting splinting is worn at all times. The athlete should attempt to run without the splint only once the ankle has been fully rehabilitated.

It is important to prevent repeated ankle injuries, as each injury increases the likelihood that the athlete will be left with a chronically unstable ankle at risk of re-injury. Thus some

Ismael Kirui (see page 120)

Interview
In December 1994, in London, I sprained my ankle while out training for a cross-country challenge event in France. My ankle was swollen, and it was extremely painful when touched, or when weight was put on it. I was forced out of running for one and a half weeks, but was able to resume light training afterwards.

I then took part in the Kenyan cross-country trials, where I placed fifth, to make sure of my place in the world championships in Durham, UK. I came third at the World Cross Challenge race in Durham, and won the Cross Challenge series for 1994–1995

Before the 1995 World Cross-Country Championships I attended a high altitude training camp in Kenya. My ankle was still sore so I just ran lightly for the first week and had more ultrasound treatment. After that I had no more problems and went on to take second place in the World Championship event.

Our comment
The inversion strain that Ismael Kirui suffered was clearly not too serious as it responded to a minimum of treatment, as do most such injuries. Most ankle strains are not sufficiently severe to prevent running. But it is important that the still-injured ankle be strapped or placed in an aircast splint for the first few weeks after an inversion injury. Some ankle injuries cause persistent problems, because of continued inflammation of the joint lining caused by the original injury. The correct treatment of this delayed complication of an otherwise minor injury is surgical removal of the inflamed tissues inside the ankle.

---

runners who have already suffered from repeated ankle sprains may benefit by using the ankle splint almost constantly, and certainly when they are running on uneven surfaces.

More severe injuries, in which there are also bone fractures or complete ligament ruptures, will require surgery.

Eversion strain

Diagnosis
In eversion strain (sprained medial ankle ligaments), pain is felt below the inner ankle bone. Swelling and bruising will discolour the foot. Forcing the foot upwards and outwards induces pain.

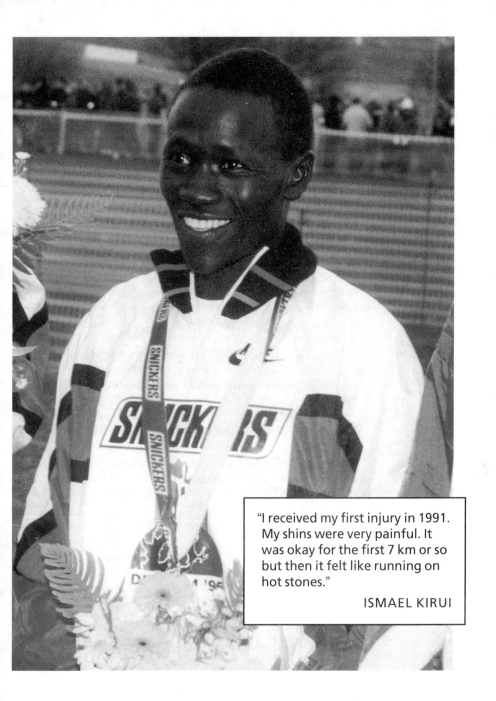

"I received my first injury in 1991. My shins were very painful. It was okay for the first 7 km or so but then it felt like running on hot stones."

ISMAEL KIRUI

A severe injury can lead to fractures of the tips (malleoli) of the fibula and tibia, with a higher fracture of the fibula also being possible. Extreme local tenderness over the bone is indicative of this, although radiological diagnosis is usually necessary to confirm this injury.

Cause
The injury is caused by turning the ankle over onto the inside of the foot, usually by running over a rock or other projecting object. This is a less common injury than the inversion strain.

Treatment
The treatment is as for the inversion strain. Again, the injury must be treated with circumspection as there may be hidden problems.

Occasionally there are delayed complications: the runner may continue to have discomfort for months after the initial injury has apparently resolved. This may be due to trapping of the joint lining (sinovium). A simple surgical procedure cures the problem.

There is also some evidence that ankle sprains which are poorly treated initially may lead to osteoarthritis in later life. For this reason, these injuries should always be treated with great care.

Stress fractures of the calcaneus, navicular and talus bones
Stress fractures of these ankle bones (see diagrams pages 145–6) are uncommon injuries and should be dealt with according to the points raised under the general discussion of stress fractures on page 68.

Diagnosis
The pain is well localized to these bones. Bone scan techniques should be used to confirm the fracture where there is diagnostic uncertainty. Even then, some fractures may not show on the bone scan.

Treatment
The only effective treatment is six weeks' rest from running.

Steve Moneghetti (see page 35)

Interview

I have twice turned over my ankle in training, both times suffering ligament damage, with the ankle swelling and turning black and blue. In 1989 I received immediate intensive treatment, in the form of icing and elevating the ankle, and using crutches to keep my weight off the foot. Further treatment included heat packs, ultrasound, cross-friction and wobbleboard exercises.

Because of the early treatment, I only missed four days of training, but in 1994, when I was five hours away from a physiotherapist when I suffered the injury, I was out of training for five days and then an additional two days when my ankle did not respond as quickly as it might have.

Paula Radcliffe (see page 76)

Interview

After my leg came out of plaster, following my stress fracture in my metatarsal in 1994, I found I had lost a lot of leg muscle. I slowly built up my training.

I had two races in June and July that year, but could hardly walk afterwards. A gait analyst diagnosed dropped arches and recommended orthotics. It was clear that my stress fracture had healed, but my foot was still stiff. I first tried rigid plastic orthotics, then a semi-flexible variety, then a fully flexible one.

After completing my second year of European studies at Loughborough University, I went to work in Germany in October. My foot still hurt and I'd still been running in the pool up to that time. In Germany, tendonitis of the tendon in my foot was diagnosed. I feel it was at least partly due to losing leg muscle when I was in plaster.

I stuck to running on grass and working out in the gym during my lunch hour. I also had physiotherapy. I ran a few races, but my foot felt very stiff after a cross-country race in Seville.

Tendonitis was again confirmed and I was treated in Germany. A lot of fluid was removed from my ankle joint and I received three injections of a natural protozoa, which broke down the scar tissue. I also took supplements of calcium and vitamins. I was also using special light orthotics and my foot felt improved.

For the first time in a year I was able to run pain-free and able to train specifically for the World Cross-Country Championships.

Stress fracture of the cuboid bone

Diagnosis
Frequently, stress fracture of the cuboid bone (see diagram page 146) over which the peroneal tendon runs, is confused with peroneus tendonitis. Unlike other stress fractures, a feature of the cuboid fracture is that it does not usually cause pain that is sufficiently severe to prevent all running. Thus the important diagnostic feature is persistent discomfort over the cuboid bone that does not resolve within three to five weeks. The injury is usually only apparent on a bone scan, not on X-rays.

Cause
The specific biomechanical cause of this injury is not known. General factors discussed in chapter six under stress fractures and relating to training errors and hereditary factors are applicable. Again, the injury is more common in those whose bones are weak for the reasons already described.

Treatment
The injury usually resolves after five to eight weeks' rest.

Tibialis posterior tendonitis and subtalar pronation syndrome

Diagnosis and cause
Tendonitis of the tibialis posterior tendon and subtalar pronation syndrome both cause pain immediately below the lower tip (medial malleolus) of the tibia. The distinction between the two conditions is of little practical importance as both are due to excessive ankle pronation and respond only to adequate control of this tendency.

Treatment
Thus the treatment is the same as that for peripatellar pain syndrome, achilles tendonitis and plantar fasciitis.

Peroneus tendonitis
Inflammation of the peroneus tendon, peroneus tendonitis, is an uncommon injury of unknown biomechanical origins. The treatment should be as for any other chronic tendon injury, notably achilles tendonitis.

Foot

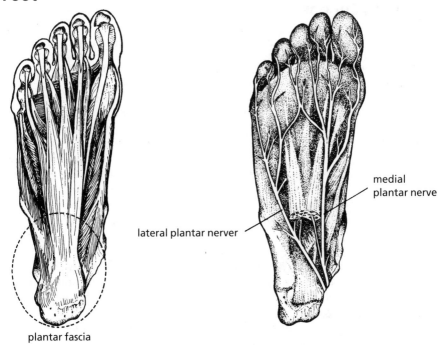

lateral plantar nerver

medial
plantar nerve

plantar fascia

Plantar fasciitis

The plantar fascia is a band which stretches across the base of
the foot, from the heel to the bases of the toes, providing a
protective covering underfoot. The site of injury is almost
always at the attachment to the heel bone (see diagram on left
above). The plantar fascia is one of the major shock-absorbing
structures of the foot.

Diagnosis

The injury presents as pain below the heel which is usually first
noticed during running, then becomes noticeable on getting up
in the morning. For the first few steps injured runners hobble by
putting all their weight on the heel and will not extend the
ankle or push off with the big toe. (The same features are present
in achilles tendonitis.) Someone suffering from a heel bruise, on
the other hand, will hobble on the toes in order to prevent the
bruised heel from coming into contact with the ground.

Gwynneth Coogan *(United States of America)*

US team-member for 1992 Olympic Games in Barcelona and for the 1993, 1994, and 1995 World Cross-Country Championships, where she placed 101st, 27th, and 37th respectively. USA 1994 national silver medallist for both 5000 m (15:39) and 10 000 m (32:08). Second place in US Cross-Country Championships in 1991, 1992 and 1994

Mother of one daughter, she is a maths lecturer and doctoral student at the University of Colorado.

Interview

I had always enjoyed team sports, such as hockey and lacrosse, but I thought I'd try something else while at college, so I started running. I did quite well, but after about two and a half years I began to experience a pain in my foot. This coincided with changing my shoes and increased mileage in my training.

Instead of cutting back or stopping, I just carried on and the pain worsened. I was under pressure at college and began to wonder whether the pain wasn't the classic 'in the head' syndrome. But the injury persisted, especially when running up and down hills. It was then diagnosed as plantar fasciitis and I started to treat the injury more conventionally through stretching, icing and massage.

I often sat with my foot in a bucket of ice. Eventually someone asked me why I was doing that and responded, 'But that's ridiculous!'. I thought to myself: 'Yes, it is!' and stopped.

Although it was an important phase in my training, I stopped running completely and 'treated' the injury successfully by cycling through Europe for two months!

Our comment   Plantar fasciitis usually requires a custom-built orthotic.

On examination, the diagnostic feature is extreme, localized tenderness at the front of the calcaneus or heel bone, where the plantar fascia attaches to that bone (see diagram page 153).

The pain may be reproduced by stretching the fascia by pulling the toes towards the knee.

Cause
The mechanism of injury in this condition is believed to be excessive ankle pronation (as for peripatellar pain syndrome),

which causes a bowstring stretching of the plantar fascia, especially if toe-off occurs with the ankle fully pronated. There is some suggestion, however, that the injury is more common in those with cavus (high-arched) feet that fail to pronate sufficiently. This suggests that inadequate shock absorption may also play an important role.

Treatment
Until the exact mechanism of this injury has been determined, treatment should include measures to stop excessive ankle pronation. Thus all the measures described for the treatment of runner's knee and achilles tendonitis must be tried. It may be necessary to adjust the corrective orthotic slightly to ensure that it does not contact the painful area under the heel bone. In fact, orthotics have been known to cause inflammation of the fascia and for this injury softer orthotics may be required.

Calf-muscle stretching (see exercise 7 and 10 on pages 51 and 52) would seem to be important both in the prevention and the cure of the injury. Uphill running (which stretches the fascia) and speedwork should be avoided until the injury has resolved.

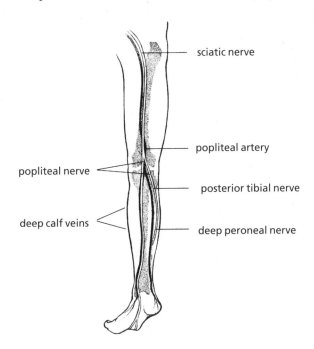

sciatic nerve

popliteal artery

popliteal nerve

posterior tibial nerve

deep calf veins

deep peroneal nerve

Eamonn Martin (see page 31)

Interview   *I had suffered plantar fasciitis twice prior to fitting the orthotics, but the injury recurred in 1993. The problem was my reluctance to use orthotics in racing. I was competing in the Europa Cup 10 000 m at Rome in 1993 in spikes without orthotics when the injury struck again. The injury was successfully treated, but this time I made sure of getting another pair of specially-made orthotics to fit the spikes. So far I have not had a recurrence of the injury.*

If this approach fails to be effective, the possibility that the injury is due to inadequate shock absorption should be considered, and the measures suggested for the treatment of the iliotibial band friction syndrome, in particular the softer running shoe, should be attempted.

In runners in whom symptoms persist for more than twelve months despite all these measures, surgery may prove very effective. In these runners the inflammation of the attachment of the plantar fascia may have set up a reaction of new bone growth on the heel bone, causing the development of a 'heel spur'. There is no evidence that the surgical removal of the heel spur is of any lasting value.

Nerve entrapment syndromes

Recently it has become apparent that a group of nerve entrapment syndromes can cause pain in the foot. Four sites have been identified in the foot where these injuries, which are resistant to all forms of conventional therapy, occur.

Diagnosis

The following are the relevant diagnostic features:

☐ Pain that is indistinguishable from the pain arising from plantar fasciitis is caused by the entrapment of the nerve to the abductor digiti quinti muscle (muscle on the outside of the foot) which runs deep into the plantar fascia.

☐ Pain on top of the foot, often radiating to the toes, is caused by the entrapment of the deep peroneal nerve as it crosses either the talus (lower ankle bone) or the tarso-metatarsal joint (see diagram page 155).

Catherina McKiernan

(see page 38)

Interview   *I received my first serious injury at the worst time — shortly before the World Track and Field Championships in 1995. My form had given me confidence for the 10 000 m, as I had beaten most of the serious competitors in the build-up races.*

I had been training at altitude at Davos, Switzerland, in June 1995, when I began to feel discomfort under my foot. I received treatment for the inflamed tendon and I continued to train on it. The injury was diagnosed as plantar fasciitis and eased with the treatment, but flared up again during the 5000 m at the Bislet Games in Oslo, Norway. Three laps into the race it flared up again. But I didn't want to drop out so I continued and my foot became progressively worse. In hindsight I should have dropped out early as continuing the race merely aggravated the injury.

Back home I immediately made plans to see a specialist in London, two weeks prior to the Championships. Intensive physiotherapy, which included cross-frictions and ultrasound, helped initially but continued frictions did not appear to improve the injury further. I rested the injury at home for a few days after that in the hope that I would be able to compete at Göteborg. Unfortunately I could not run freely, and had to withdraw.

Our comment   Certain injuries, like achilles tendonitis, (see Elana Meyer on page 135) and plantar fasciitis, seem to occur more frequently in elite athletes who have trained at high intensity for many years. Perhaps these tendons or ligaments are less able than muscles and bones to accommodate, adapt to, or recover from the stresses of frequent, high intensity, eccentric loadings.

The long-term use of a corrective orthotic will most likely reduce the risk of frequent re-injury in runners prone to plantar fascia or achilles tendon injuries. It is possible that had McKiernan been fitted with an appropriate orthotic as soon as the plantar fascia injury occurred, she may have been able to compete at Göteborg.

☐ Pain is felt on the lower surface of the foot as well as on the inside of the heel owing to the entrapment of the posterior tibial nerve (see diagram page 155).

☐ Pain is felt on the inside of the foot, just above and in front of the site at which the plantar fascia is tender in runners with plantar fasciitis.

This is due to the entrapment of the medial plantar nerve below the joint between the calcaneus (heel bone) and the navicular (see diagram page 153).

Cause
The cause of these entrapments is unknown.

Treatment
Surgical decompression of these nerves at the site of entrapment is the only effective form of treatment. As these are unusual injuries, they will usually be diagnosed only by those who are experienced in the treatment of running injuries.

Stress fracture of the metatarsals

Diagnosis
Stress fractures of the metatarsals or toe bones cause severe pain that prevents running. The pain can be reproduced by pressing the injured metatarsal from above. Other diagnostic characteristics are discussed under stress fractures on page 68.

Cause
The causes of stress fractures in general, as discussed on page 71, are applicable here. Usually the injury relates to an increase in training distance or running on a harder surface. Two groups especially at risk in this injury are female runners who start training too hard and runners who have rigid feet and run in hard running shoes. Often the bone affected will be determined by running style. Thus the third or fourth metatarsal could fracture in runners tending to run on the outside of their feet, while the second metatarsal is at risk in those runners who pronate.

Treatment
The treatment is six weeks' rest from running. When the bone is no longer sore to the touch running may be resumed, but a gradual build-up to fitness is advised.

Gwynneth Coogan (see page 154)

Interview   *I was training hard for the 1992 World Cross-Country Championships, as they were to be held in my home town of Boston. The injury seemed to come out of nowhere, but I think the problem was compensating for hurting my foot in running cross-country.*

A bone scan confirmed a fracture of the third metatarsal, just four weeks prior to the cross-country trial for the world championships. I ran in water and biked a lot and my foot felt okay just before the trial. But in the end I decided not to risk it as the Olympic trials were just a few months off. So I rested it a week or two more and fortunately made the team to Barcelona.

Our comment   Stress fractures of the foot usually heal within five to six weeks, during which time the athlete needs to consider why the injury occurred and how further fractures can be prevented. The role of diet and menstruation must be considered in young women.

Digital neuritis

Diagnosis
Pain on the top of the foot could be similar to the pain found in stress fracture except that it is less severe and hinders, rather than prevents, running. There may be pain down the toes.

Cause
This injury is caused by pressure from the shoe upper, in particular from the shoe laces, on the small digital nerves as they run over the bony prominences on the back of the foot. Shoes with the D-ring lacing system or other systems with rigid, plastic eyelets for the laces may be particularly liable to cause this injury.

Treatment
The treatment is to isolate the site at which the nerve is tender and alter the shoe lacing so that no laces cause pressure there.

If altering the lacing pattern does not cure the injury, some form of padding, for example Spenco material, should be glued to the back of the shoe tongue to protect the site of pain.

Digital neuroma

Diagnosis
This injury causes marked, well-localized pain under the affected metatarsal. The pain becomes progressively worse the further the athlete runs. The most important diagnostic feature is a tender knot of nerve and scar tissue, about the size of half a peanut, that causes a distinct, painful click as it is rolled from side to side over the head of the nearest metatarsal. The pain is relieved by stopping running and removing the shoe.

Cause
In digital neuroma, one of the small nerves on the bottom of the foot becomes inflamed, hard and tender as a result of compression between the metatarsal bones and the mid-sole of the running shoe.

Treatment
If the condition is not severe it may be eased by a pad placed directly behind the affected metatarsal bone, which will prevent the nerve being caught between the metatarsal and the shoe. Otherwise the only treatment is surgical removal of the neuroma.

Metatarsal trauma

Diagnosis
Metatarsal trauma or metatarsalgia causes more diffuse pain, which spreads across two or more of the metatarsal bones.

Cause
This injury is due to excessive landing pressure on the bones of a foot which is biomechanically imbalanced (often an excessively high-arched foot) so that landing force is localized to these bones, rather than distributed across all the bones of the forefoot.

Treatment
The treatment is to use softer running shoes with a Spenco or Sorbothane insole to absorb additional shock. Should that fail, an orthopaedic technician should be consulted to apply what is known as a metatarsal bar to the outside of the shoe immediately behind the ball of the foot. Alternatively, a corrective orthotic should be used in an attempt to distribute landing

Antonio Pinto (see page 46)

Interview

In January 1995, I suffered a sharp pain at the top of my foot, which kept me from training for a few days. The cause and treatment were simple: my orthotic insert was too high and caused too much pressure from my shoe upper. I simply replaced it with a lower one and the problem disappeared.

forces more evenly across the foot. Usually these measures cure the injury, but they may require some months of adjustment before they are totally effective.

The possibility of a nerve entrapment syndrome should be considered when chronic foot pain persists despite treatment.

Black toenails

Diagnosis
The nail starts to turn black near the base.

Cause
These can be caused by a single blow, but more often black toenails are the result of the toenail catching the inner shoe lining as the foot hits the ground, and the toes move downwards inside the shoe to touch the ground. The rubbing between the toes and the shoe causes a lifting force on the toenails, which causes the nail to bleed at its base and turn black.

Treatment
The pressure can be relieved by boring through the nail with a heated pin or paper clip, allowing the trapped blood to be released. Toenails should be kept trimmed and shoe selection should take into account the above factors. If problems persist a chiropodist or podiatrist should be consulted. Black toenails should be removed. The condition can be prevented by cutting the front of the shoe (the toe-box) where the upper attaches to the mid-sole in the region of the toes.

Diagnosis chart

This chart is intended as a starting point on the path towards a diagnosis. The page numbers on the right hand side indicate where a detailed discussion of each injury may be found.

Upper torso and buttocks	1 Stitch	■ Severe pain on right side of abdomen below rib margin ■ Pain only during exercise ■ Pain often felt in right shoulder joint	90
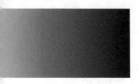	2 Sciatica	■ Pain shoots from back through buttocks, possibly to feet ■ Pain felt when lifting leg while lying face-up	92
	3 Chronic muscle tears	■ Discomfort in buttock while running ■ Localized tenderness ■ Tender knot can be located by applying finger pressure at site of pain	95

Hip, pelvis and groin	1 Chronic tears of adductor muscle	■ Pain begins gradually, worsens with continued exercise ■ Pain subsides with rest but recurs immediately on running ■ Tender knot felt on palpation of painful site	97
	2 Chronic tears of psoas muscle	■ Onset of pain gradual ■ Pain passes off with rest but recurs during exercise ■ Pain reproduced by lying face-up and flexing knee against resistance ■ Tender knot felt on palpation of painful site	98
	3 Stress fracture of pelvis	■ Initial discomfort in groin ■ Pain worsens to point where running becomes impossible ■ Runner cannot stand on injured leg alone	98

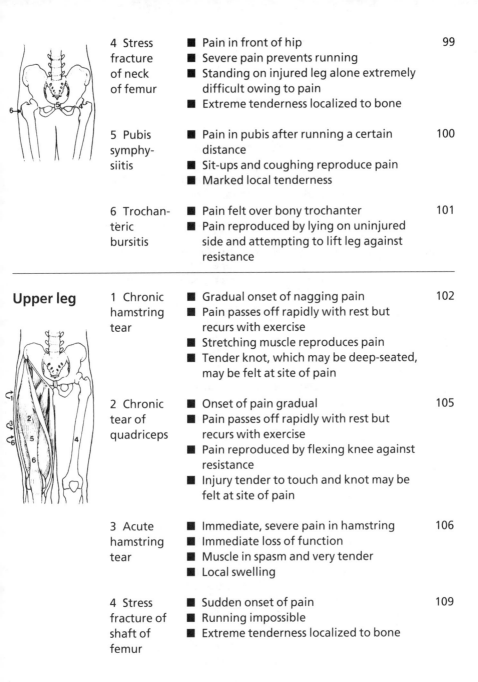

	4 Stress fracture of neck of femur	■ Pain in front of hip ■ Severe pain prevents running ■ Standing on injured leg alone extremely difficult owing to pain ■ Extreme tenderness localized to bone	99
	5 Pubis symphysiitis	■ Pain in pubis after running a certain distance ■ Sit-ups and coughing reproduce pain ■ Marked local tenderness	100
	6 Trochanteric bursitis	■ Pain felt over bony trochanter ■ Pain reproduced by lying on uninjured side and attempting to lift leg against resistance	101

Upper leg

	1 Chronic hamstring tear	■ Gradual onset of nagging pain ■ Pain passes off rapidly with rest but recurs with exercise ■ Stretching muscle reproduces pain ■ Tender knot, which may be deep-seated, may be felt at site of pain	102
	2 Chronic tear of quadriceps	■ Onset of pain gradual ■ Pain passes off rapidly with rest but recurs with exercise ■ Pain reproduced by flexing knee against resistance ■ Injury tender to touch and knot may be felt at site of pain	105
	3 Acute hamstring tear	■ Immediate, severe pain in hamstring ■ Immediate loss of function ■ Muscle in spasm and very tender ■ Local swelling	106
	4 Stress fracture of shaft of femur	■ Sudden onset of pain ■ Running impossible ■ Extreme tenderness localized to bone	109

	5 Delayed muscle soreness of quadriceps and hamstring	■ Muscle pain peaks 24 to 48 hours after exercise	109
	6 Muscle cramping of quadriceps and hamstring	■ Spasmodic, involuntary, painful contraction of muscle ■ Often associated with unaccustomed distance or speed	109

Knee	1 Peripatellar pain syndrome ('runner's knee')	■ Pain localized around kneecap, usually at lower end ■ Pain usually begins after running a predictable distance ■ Walking up or down stairs causes discomfort ■ Sitting with knee bent causes discomfort	110
	2 Iliotibial band friction syndrome (ITB)	■ Severe pain localized over outside of knee ■ Site tender to pressure ■ Pain felt only during exercise	113
	3 Osgood-Schlatter syndrome	■ Specific to growing children ■ Discomfort localized over tibial tubercle (knob below knee)	118
	4 Chronic tears of vastus medialis muscles	■ Onset of pain gradual ■ Pain passes off with rest but recurs with exercise ■ Pain reproduced by lying face-up and flexing knee against resistance ■ Tender knot may be felt at site of pain	119
	5 Popliteus tendonitis	■ Pain on outside of knee just below site where ITB causes pain ■ Gradual onset of pain ■ Pain worsens with continued exercise	121

Lower leg

1 Posterior and anterior tibial bone strain ('shin-splints')	■ Initial vague pain in calf after exercise ■ As training continues, pain comes on during exercise ■ Pain eventually becomes extreme during exercise ■ Tenderness localized to back of or front border of tibia	121
2 Fibular bone strain ('shin-splints')	■ Initial vague pain in calf after exercise ■ As training continues, pain comes on during exercise ■ Pain eventually becomes extreme during exercise ■ Tenderness localized to outside edge of fibula	121
3 Stress fracture of tibia	■ Injury occurs suddenly without external trauma ■ Running impossible ■ Extreme tenderness localized to bone ■ Hopping on injured leg painful or impossible	126
4 Stress fracture of fibula	■ Injury occurs suddenly without external trauma ■ Diagnosis difficult as injury may not prevent running ■ Tenderness localized over fibula	127
5 Chronic tears of calf muscles	■ Discomfort localized to calf muscles ■ Onset of pain gradual but worsens with continued exercise ■ Pain passes off quickly with rest but injury is not cured without cross-frictions ■ May be difficult to push off strongly with ankle on affected side	129
6 Chronic tear of anterior tibial muscle	■ Muscle exquisitely tender at injured site ■ Knot may be felt at site of pain ■ Pain felt by flexing ankle against resistance	130

7 Chronic tear of posterior tibial muscle	■ Muscle exquisitely tender at injured site ■ Knot at injured site may be deep-seated, under main calf muscle ■ Pain reproduced by pushing foot and toes down hard against resistance while turning foot inwards	130
8 Delayed muscle soreness of calf muscles	■ Muscle pain peaks 24 to 48 hours after exercise	131
9 Cramping of calf muscles	■ Spasmodic, painful, involuntary contraction of muscle ■ Onset common over unaccustomed distance or speed	131
10 Chronic compart-ment syndrome	■ Onset of pain during or after exercise ■ Pain worsens with continued training ■ As muscles become painful they become board-hard ■ Hardness dissipates as pain subsides	131
11 Acute compart-ment syndrome	■ Usually occurs in undertrained runners ■ Sudden onset of pain in muscles after a single exercise session ■ Pain intensifies dramatically ■ Muscles become board-hard ■ Pulse in foot disappears	133
12 Achilles tendonitis	■ Exquisite tenderness is one or more areas when tendon is pinched ■ Initial discomfort on rising from bed in morning ■ Discomfort eventually during and after exercise	134
13 Partial or complete tear of achilles tendon	■ Sudden dramatic pain and weakness in ankle ■ May be possible to feel complete gap in the tendon ■ Normal walking impossible	141

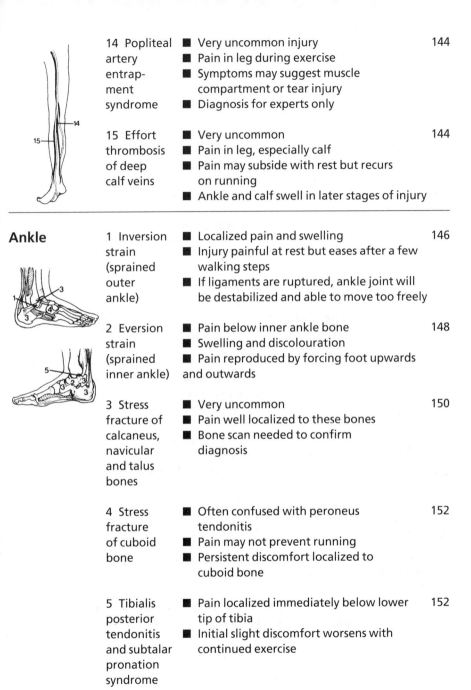

	14 Popliteal artery entrapment syndrome	■ Very uncommon injury ■ Pain in leg during exercise ■ Symptoms may suggest muscle compartment or tear injury ■ Diagnosis for experts only	144
	15 Effort thrombosis of deep calf veins	■ Very uncommon ■ Pain in leg, especially calf ■ Pain may subside with rest but recurs on running ■ Ankle and calf swell in later stages of injury	144

Ankle

	1 Inversion strain (sprained outer ankle)	■ Localized pain and swelling ■ Injury painful at rest but eases after a few walking steps ■ If ligaments are ruptured, ankle joint will be destabilized and able to move too freely	146
	2 Eversion strain (sprained inner ankle)	■ Pain below inner ankle bone ■ Swelling and discolouration ■ Pain reproduced by forcing foot upwards and outwards	148
	3 Stress fracture of calcaneus, navicular and talus bones	■ Very uncommon ■ Pain well localized to these bones ■ Bone scan needed to confirm diagnosis	150
	4 Stress fracture of cuboid bone	■ Often confused with peroneus tendonitis ■ Pain may not prevent running ■ Persistent discomfort localized to cuboid bone	152
	5 Tibialis posterior tendonitis and subtalar pronation syndrome	■ Pain localized immediately below lower tip of tibia ■ Initial slight discomfort worsens with continued exercise	152

Foot

1 Plantar fasciitis	■ Pain below heel ■ Pain first felt while running, then on getting up in morning ■ Extreme, localized tenderness at front of heel bone	153
2 Nerve entrapment syndromes	■ Various nerves may be affected ■ Pain similar to that of plantar fasciitis ■ Pain may be on top of foot, radiating to toes ■ Pain may be on lower surface of foot, as well as inside of heel ■ Pain may be inside foot, just above and in front of site of tenderness in plantar fasciitis	156
3 Stress fracture of metatarsal bones	■ Sudden onset of severe pain ■ Running impossible ■ Pain reproduced by pressing injured metatarsal from above	158
4 Digital neuritis	■ Pain on top of foot similar to but less severe than pain of stress fractures ■ Running hindered but not prevented ■ Pain may radiate to toes	159
5 Digital neuroma	■ Pain well localized under affected metatarsal ■ Pain worsens with exercise ■ Small tender knot causes painful click when rolled over nearest metatarsal ■ Pain relieved by stopping running and removing shoe	160
6 Metatarsal trauma	■ Diffuse pain which spreads across two or more metatarsal bones	160
7 Black toenails	■ Nail starts to turn black near base ■ Some swelling possible around joint	161

Glossary

Abduction The movement of a limb or body part towards the midline of the body.

Acute A condition that has been present for a short time, usually less than three days.

Amenorrhoea The absence of menstrual periods for more than three months in a person who has previously menstruated (secondary amenorrhoea), or the failure to commence regular menstruation at the appropriate age of between 11 and 16 years (primary amenorrhoea).

Anterior The front or towards the front (of the body).

Articular cartilage The specialized cartilage that lines the ends of the bones where they form joints.

Articulation The movement that occurs between the bones inside the joints of the body.

Belly breathing Breathing that emphasizes the use of the diaphragm, rather than the intercostal (chest) muscles.

Biomechanics The mechanics of body movements.

Blood vessels The arteries, capillaries and veins that carry the blood that is pumped by the heart to the body tissues and organs.

Bones The tissues that make up the skeleton.

Bone scan The use of a radiological marker which is injected into the blood stream. The marker is taken up by bone cells that are highly active because they are either repairing a fracture or because they are responding to high loading stresses, for example at the site of a bone stress injury.

Bursae Fluid-filled sacs that are found at sites where tendons pass directly over bone. Overlying the bones, the bursae prevent damage to the tendons by reducing friction. When a bursa becomes inflamed, the condition is known as bursitis (of the named bursa).

Cardiovascular Pertaining to the heart and circulation.

Cartilage Usually used to describe the menisci of the knee (knee cartilages). The menisci are tough, fibrous structures that are attached to the articular cartilage at the top of the tibia (shin bone) where it articulates with the thigh bone, the femur.

Chronic A condition that has been present for more than a specified time, usually more than three weeks, is described as chronic.

Concentric loading Loading the muscle so that it undergoes a concentric contraction in which the muscle shortens in length as it contracts.

Concentric muscle contraction The form of muscle contraction in which the muscle shortens during the contraction.

Concentric muscle strengthening Strengthening the muscle with training techniques that use concentric muscle contractions.

Cross-frictions A specialized physiotherapeutic technique in which the muscle or tendon, usually at the site of a chronic muscle tear, is massaged sideways across the bone.

Degeneration Replacement of a localized or focal area of normal tissue, for example muscle, tendon or ligament, with damaged (scar) tissue.

Demineralization Usually used to describe a process in which the mineral content of the bones is reduced. Occurs during the early stages of running training prior to the process in which the mineral content of the bones begins to increase. Demineralization occurs with age in both men and women but increases with inactivity. Menstrual irregularity at any age is a potent cause of bone demineralization. The condition of advanced bone demineralization is known as osteoporosis.

Eccentric loading Loading the muscle so that it undergoes an eccentric contraction in which the muscle lengthens as it contracts.

Eccentric muscle contraction The form of

muscle contraction in which the muscle lengthens during the contraction.

Eccentric muscle strengthening Strengthening the muscle with training techniques that use eccentric muscle contractions.

Epiphysis The area at the ends of the bones from which bone growth occurs.

EVA Shock absorbing material (ethyl vinyl acetic acid) from which the mid-soles of most running shoes are now manufactured. First developed in the mid-1970s in the US. Prior to the development of EVA, the mid-soles of running shoes were manufactured from materials with an inadequate shock-absorbing capacity. In that it increased the shock-absorption of running shoes, the development of EVA was probably the single most important factor in improving the safety of running and thereby promoting the dramatic growth of the sport after 1976.

Extrinsic injury Injury to the human body caused by factors external to the body, for example, by an object such as a cricket ball, or another human body, as in a rugby tackle.

Flexion Bending of a joint.

Heel counter The rear section of the running shoe that surrounds the heel. This area is usually strengthened to reduce the degree to which the ankle (subtalar) joint can move during the stance phase of running.

Intrinsic injury Injury to the body that is not caused by the action of an external force on the body. Intrinsic injuries typically occur in non-contact sports like running, aerobics, etc.

Inverse stretch reflex A reflex that is activated whenever a tendon is loaded to near its breakpoint. The reflex travels from the tendon to the spinal cord where it causes inhibition of the contraction of the muscle from which the affected tendon arises.

Knot A descriptive term usually used to describe a chronic muscle tear. Palpation of the muscle reveals a painful hard area in the muscle, the muscle knot.

Lateral To the outside of the body.

Ligaments The tissues that join bones together at joints.

Loaded muscle A muscle that contracts against a load.

Medial Towards the midline of the body.

Mid-sole The mid portion of the sole of the running shoe, immediately beneath the outer sole.

Muscle cramps A condition in which one or more muscles go into painful, sustained contractions. Usually occurs during or after prolonged exercise.

Muscle fibres The individual cells which make up muscle tissue. There are two predominant types of muscle fibres or cells, the fast and slow twitch muscle fibres. Generally, long distance runners have a preponderance of slow twitch muscle fibres whereas the fast twitch fibres predominate in sprinters.

Muscles The specialized tissues attached to the bones of the skeleton that contract to produce movement.

Musculo-skeletal Pertaining to the muscles and skeleton. Usually refers to the locomotor function of the body.

Nerves The specialized tissues that convey information in the form of electrical impulses to and from the brain to all the other organs in the body.

Orthotic An in-shoe device that compensates for biomechanical abnormalities in the runner's lower limb. Orthotics are professionally made by podiatrists.

Osteoarthritis A condition in which there is destruction of the articular cartilage in one or more joints. Destruction leads to painful bone-on-bone articulation. In the sporting population, previous joint surgery following a sports-related joint injury is the commonest cause of osteoarthritis.

Osteoblasts The specialized cells that produce bone.

Osteoclasts The specialized cells that remove bone.

Osteoclonal excavation Removal of bone by the action of the osteoclasts. Bone is a dynamic organ that undergoes simultaneous production and removal. In youth, the rate of bone formation by the osteoblasts exceeds the rate of bone removal by the osteoclasts so that there is a net increase in the bone mass; after middle age, the reverse applies.

Overstriding Running with a stride that is too long. The result is that the foot must be accelerated backwards to contact the ground. Normally, the foot strikes the ground with zero acceleration in either the back- or forward direction.

Pneumatic brace A brace made from pockets of encapsulated air that surround and support the ankle or knee, thereby preventing abnormal movement of the joint.

Podiatry The profession that specializes in the management of conditions affecting the feet.

Posterior The back, or towards the back, of the body.

Pronation, including subtalar joint (rearfoot) pronation and maximum rate of pronation A complex inward and downward movement of the ankle joint. This movement allows the foot to accommodate to the surface immediately after heelstrike in the early segment of the stance phase of the running cycle. The maximum rate at which this movement occurs is termed the maximum rate of pronation.

Rupture A break in continuity of (usually) a tendon or muscle.

Skeletal Relating to the skeleton.

Sorbothane A material designed to reduce shock. It is usually used as an insole, placed inside the running shoe.

Spasm A continuous contraction of a muscle or muscle group. The same as a muscle cramp.

Spenco Commercial name to describe a shock-absorbing material developed by the American inventor, Dr Spencer, for use as an in-sole in running shoes. The development of this patented product considerably increased the wealth of this former medical practitioner. As his wealth mounted, Dr Spencer apparently demanded that each member of his family must complete a marathon race before he or she could inherit their apportioned share of his wealth.

Stance phase of the running cycle The segment of the running cycle when one foot is on the ground.

Stretch receptors Specialized tissues in the muscle, tendon or ligament that detect a change in the length of the structure.

Swing phase of the running cycle The segment of the running cycle when both feet are in the air.

Tear A break in the continuity of a muscle, tendon or ligament. Usually used to describe a small tear as opposed to a large rupture.

Tendons The specialized tissues that attach the ends of muscles to the bones on which the muscles pull to produce movement.

Thrombosis Development of a blood clot in either the arteries (arterial thrombosis) or in the veins (venous thrombosis). Arterial thrombosis leads to death of the tissues that are supplied by that artery. Venous thrombosis usually occurs in the leg veins and can lead to serious complications should sections of the clot break free and circulate through the venous circulation, coming to rest in the lung arteries and causing the death of lung tissue.

Unloaded muscle A muscle that is not subjected to any loading.

Index

Alphabetical order is letter-by-letter rather than word-by-word. Page references in **bold** refer to main treatment of a subject; those in *italic* refer to illustrations and photographs. Page references followed by *bis* indicate that there are two separate references on the page. Refer to Chapter 7 in the Contents (pages 5–7) or the Diagnosis chart (pages 162–8) for specific parts of the body.